To the amazing medical professionals, infectious disease specialists, biologists and scientists who advised me when creating this book.

Christina. Anushka. Megna. Helen. Michelle. Edna. Panna. Amy & Mike

Thank you!

For more books visit www.lycheepress.com

ISBN 978-1-953281-85-2

How do VACCINES work?

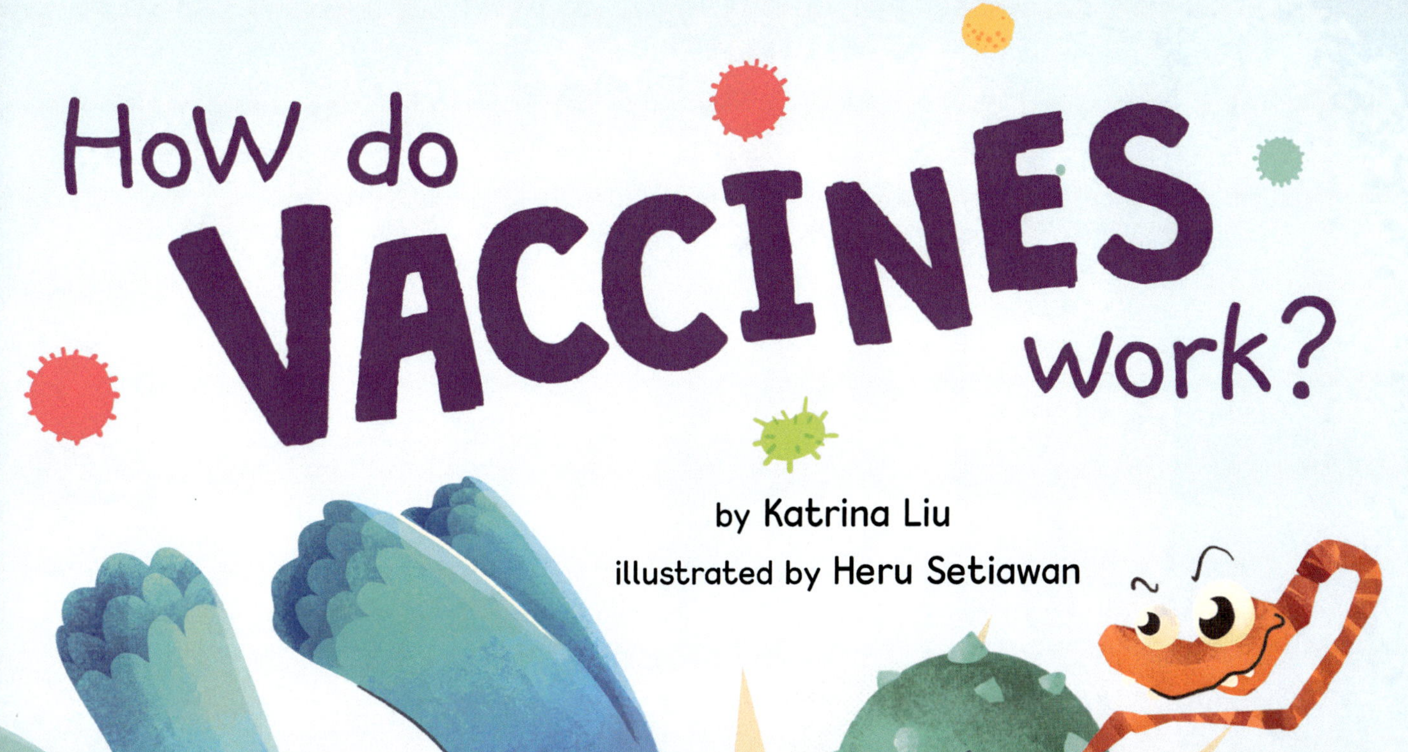

by Katrina Liu

illustrated by Heru Setiawan

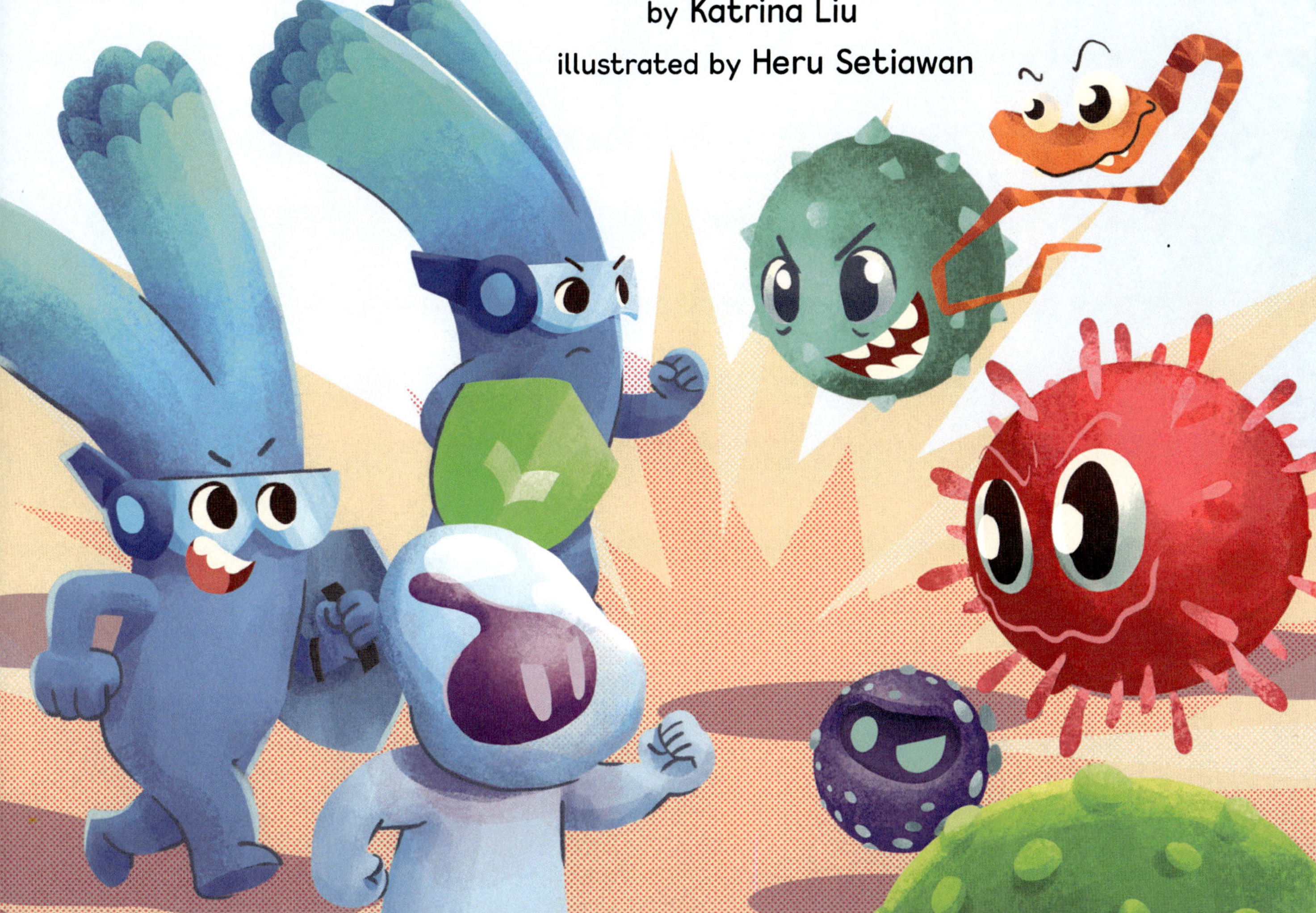

Daddy, I don't want to go to the doctor. They're going to give me a shot and shots hurt!

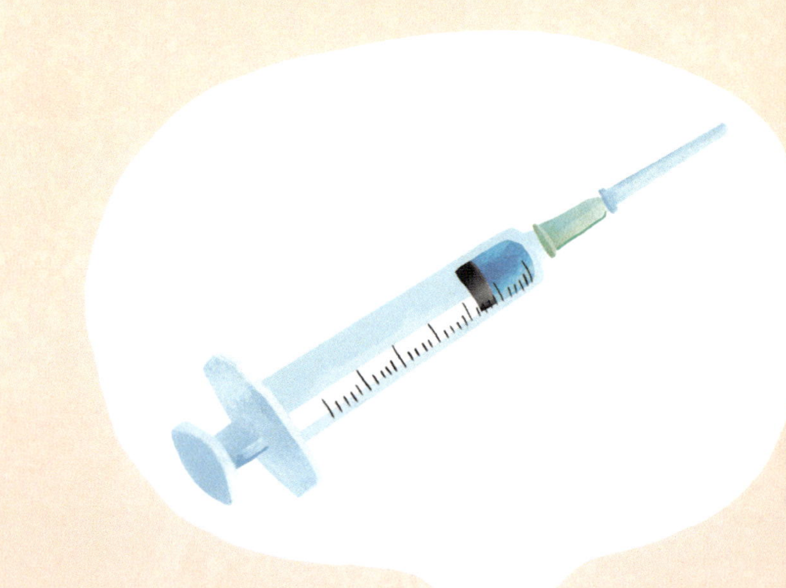

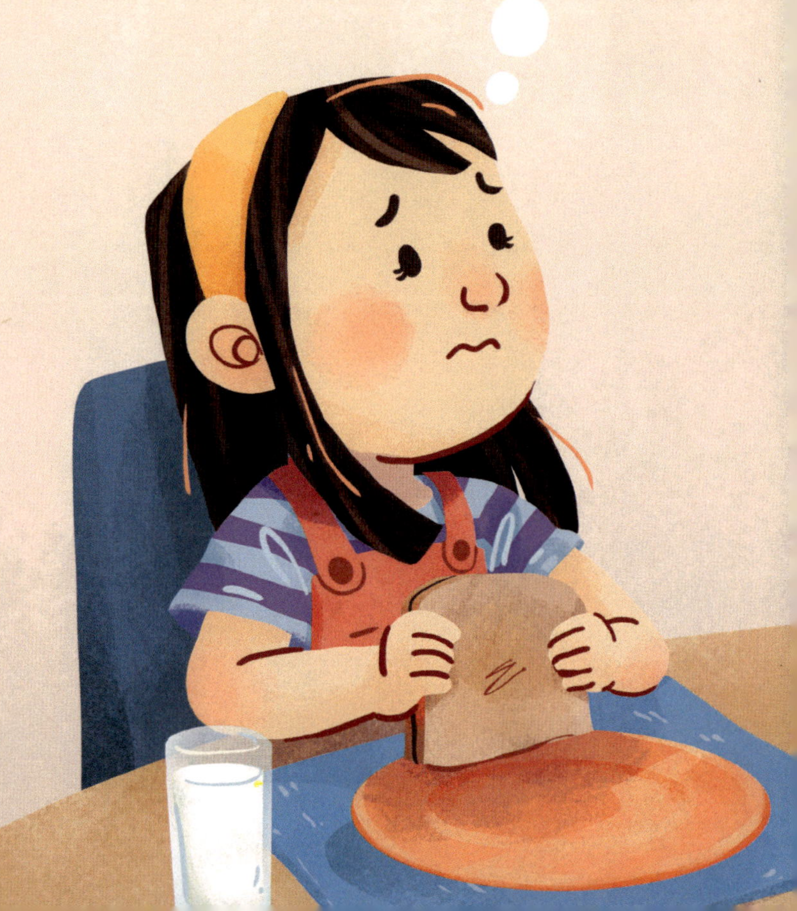

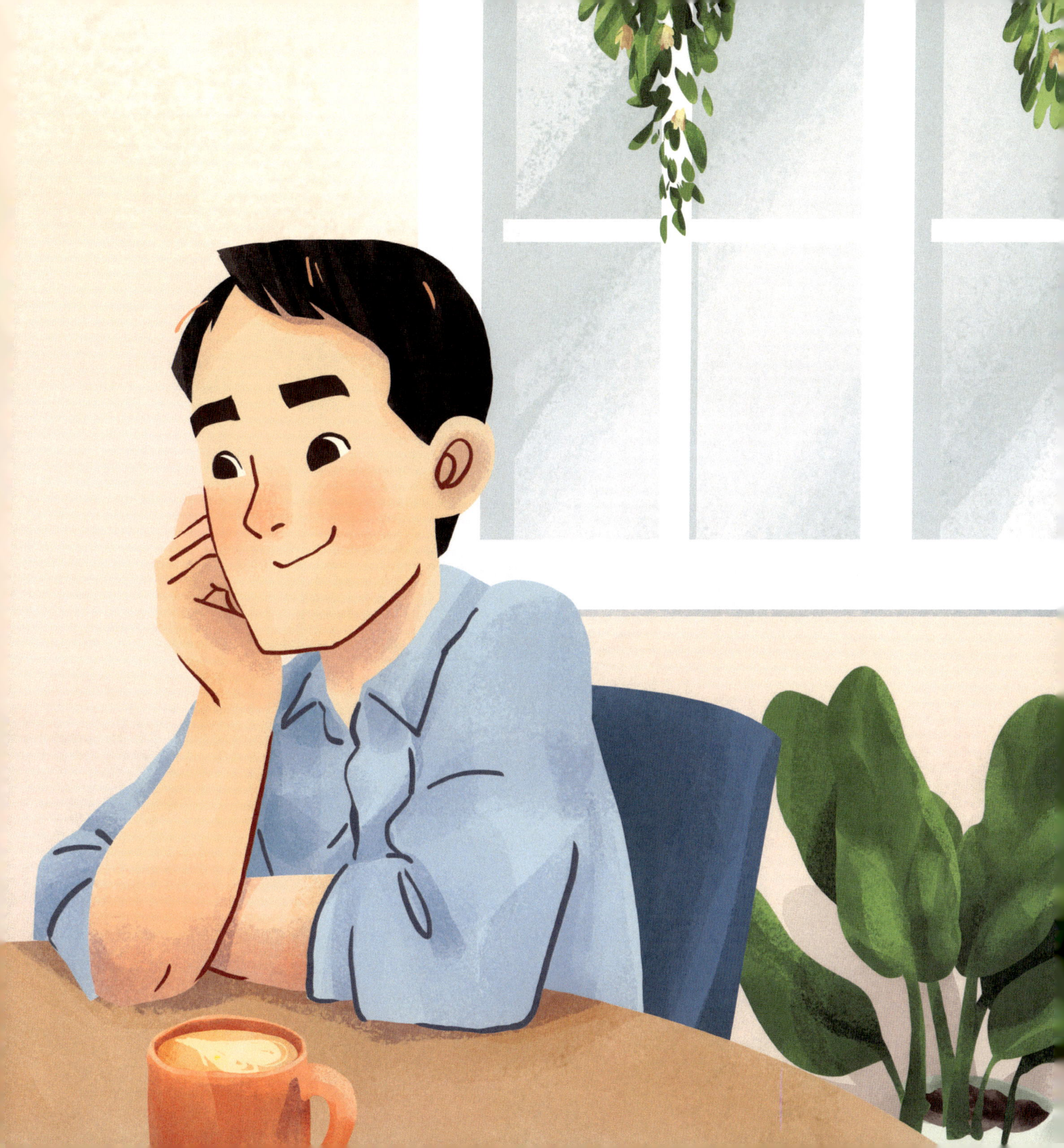

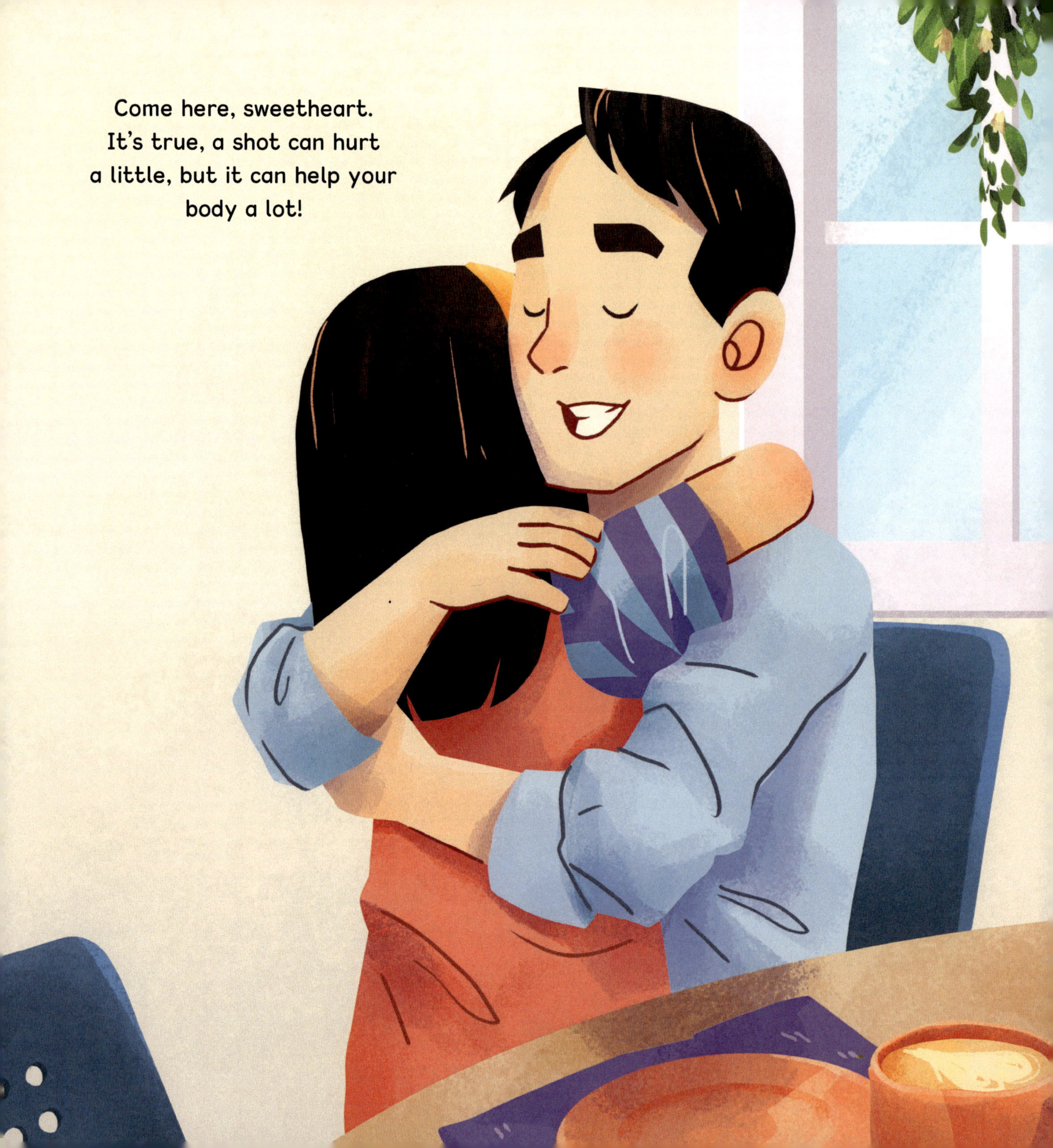
Come here, sweetheart.
It's true, a shot can hurt
a little, but it can help your
body a lot!

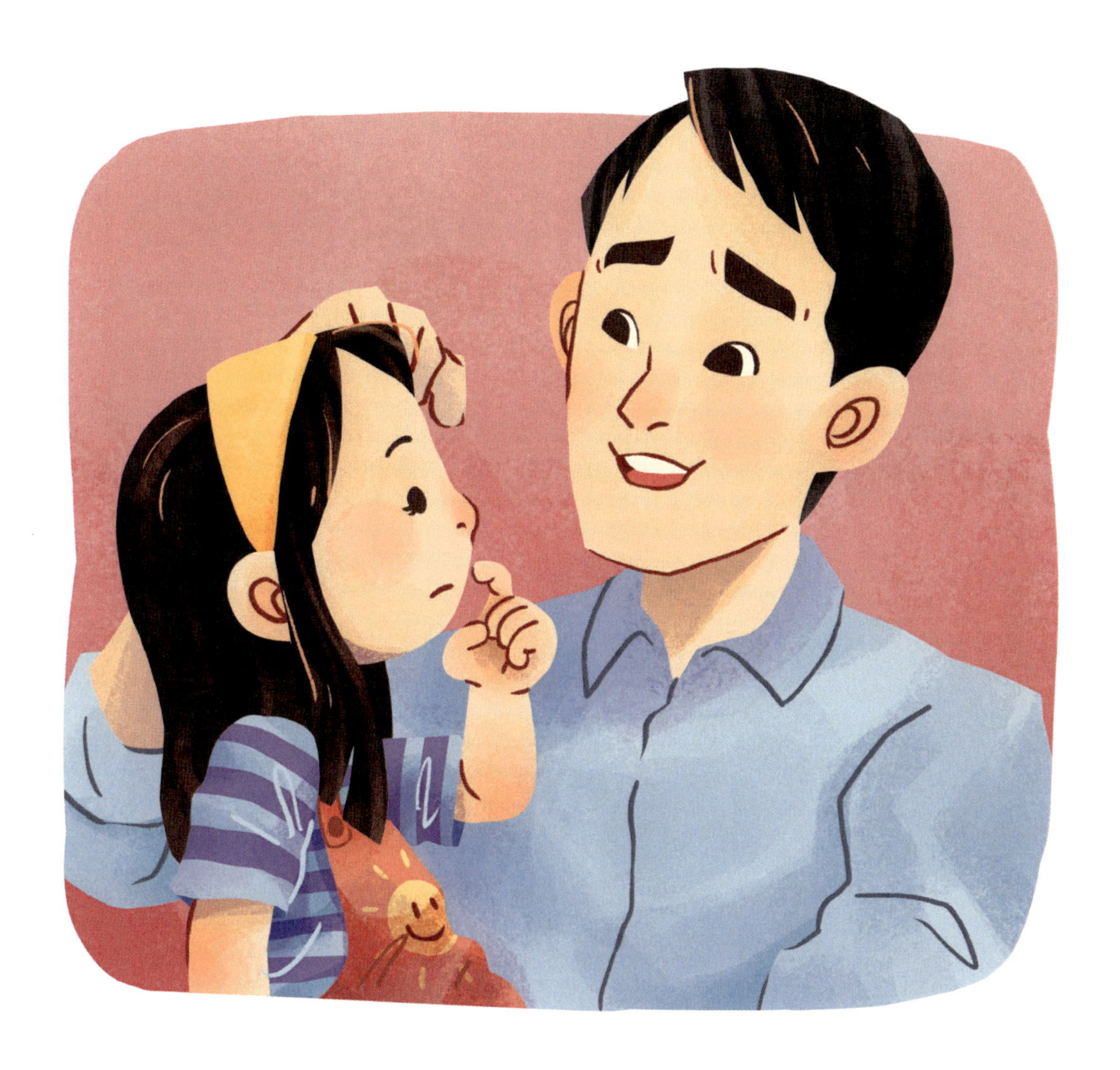

Whenever I'm scared of something, I like to learn
more about it. That helps me feel less scared.
Let me tell you how they work.

Getting a shot helps protect us from germs.

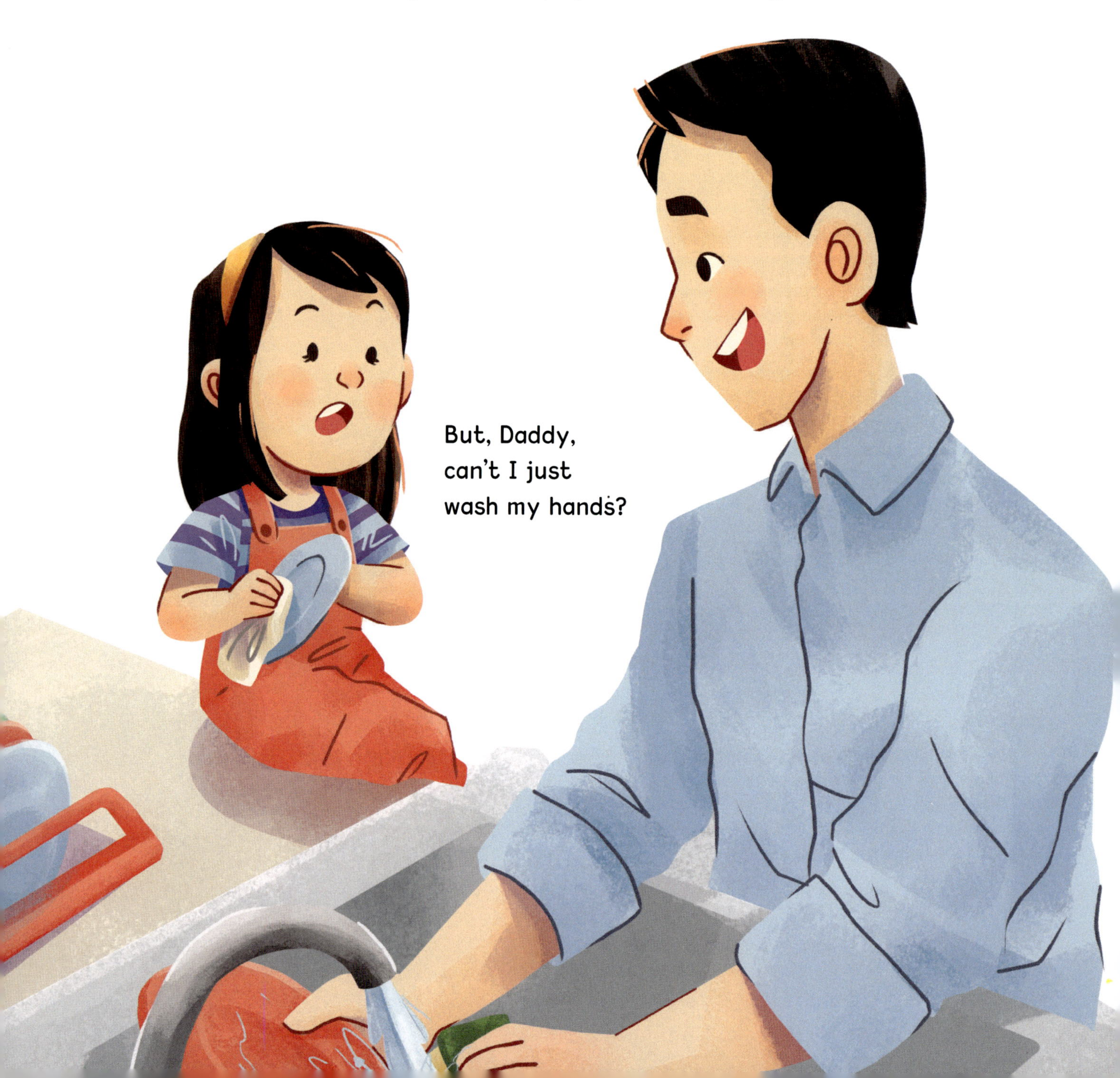

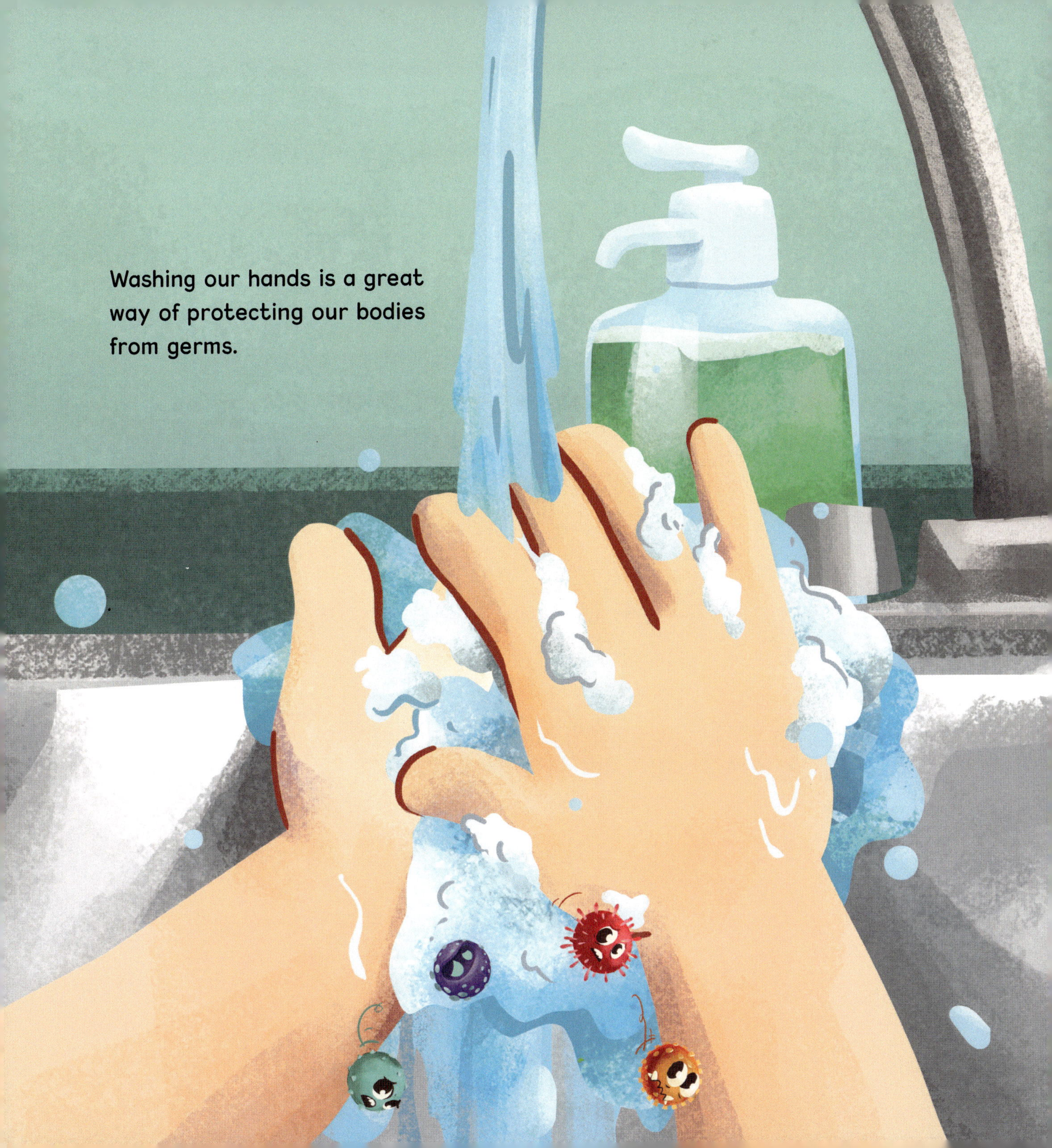

Washing our hands is a great way of protecting our bodies from germs.

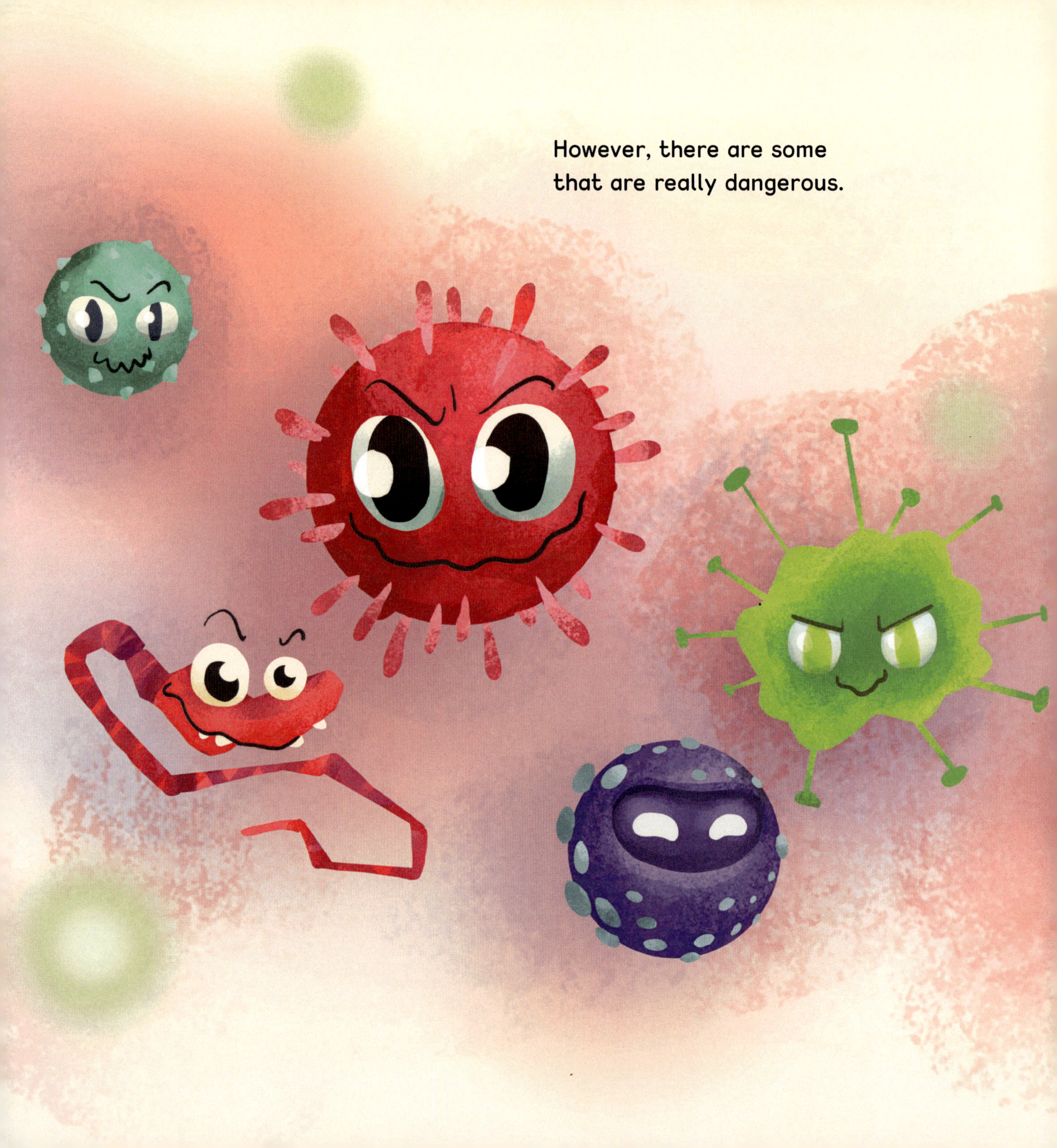

However, there are some
that are really dangerous.

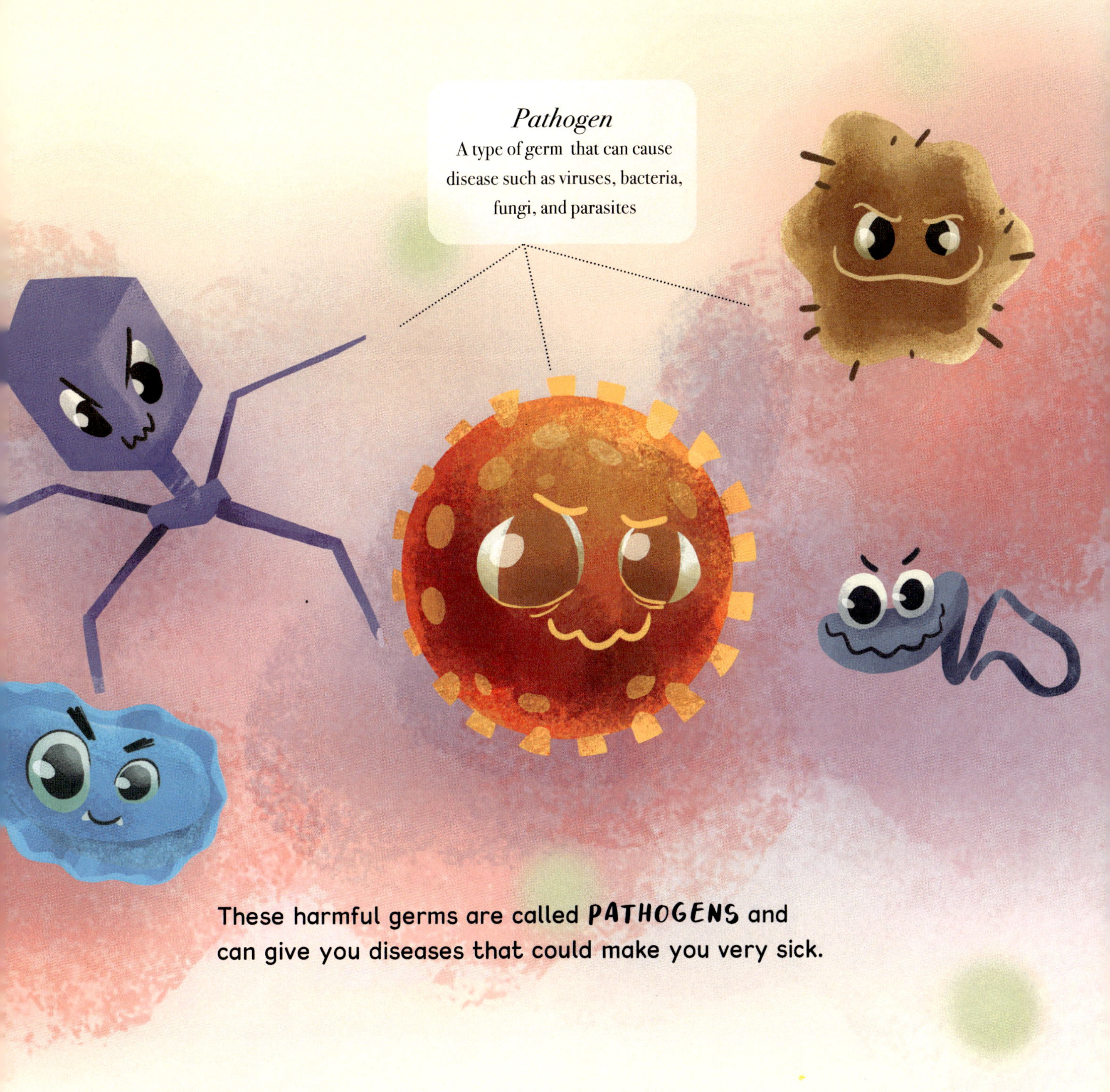

These harmful germs are called **PATHOGENS** and can give you diseases that could make you very sick.

That's why we have medicines called **VACCINES**. Sometimes they are called immunizations or shots. They give our bodies extra protection to fight off all kinds of diseases.

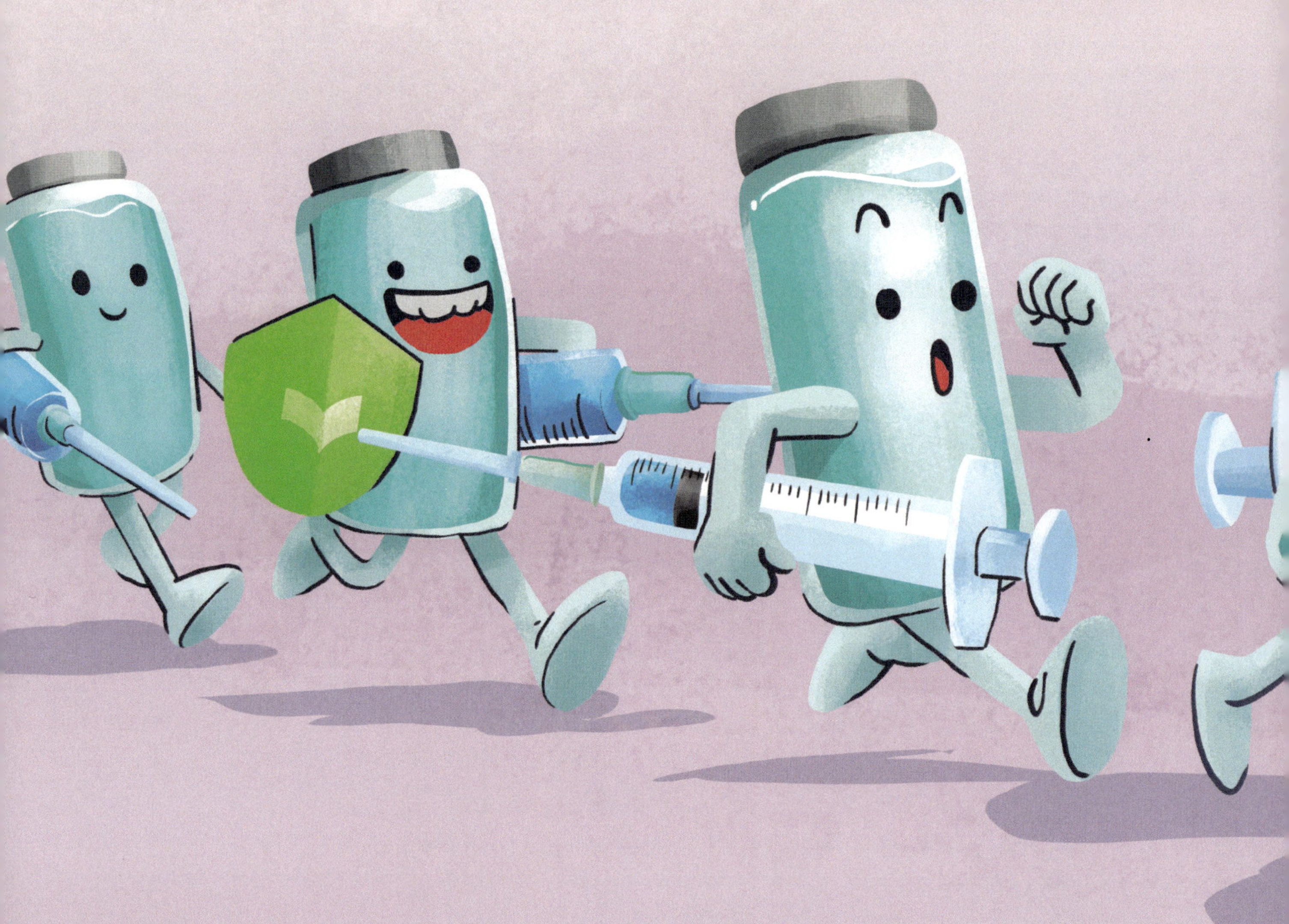

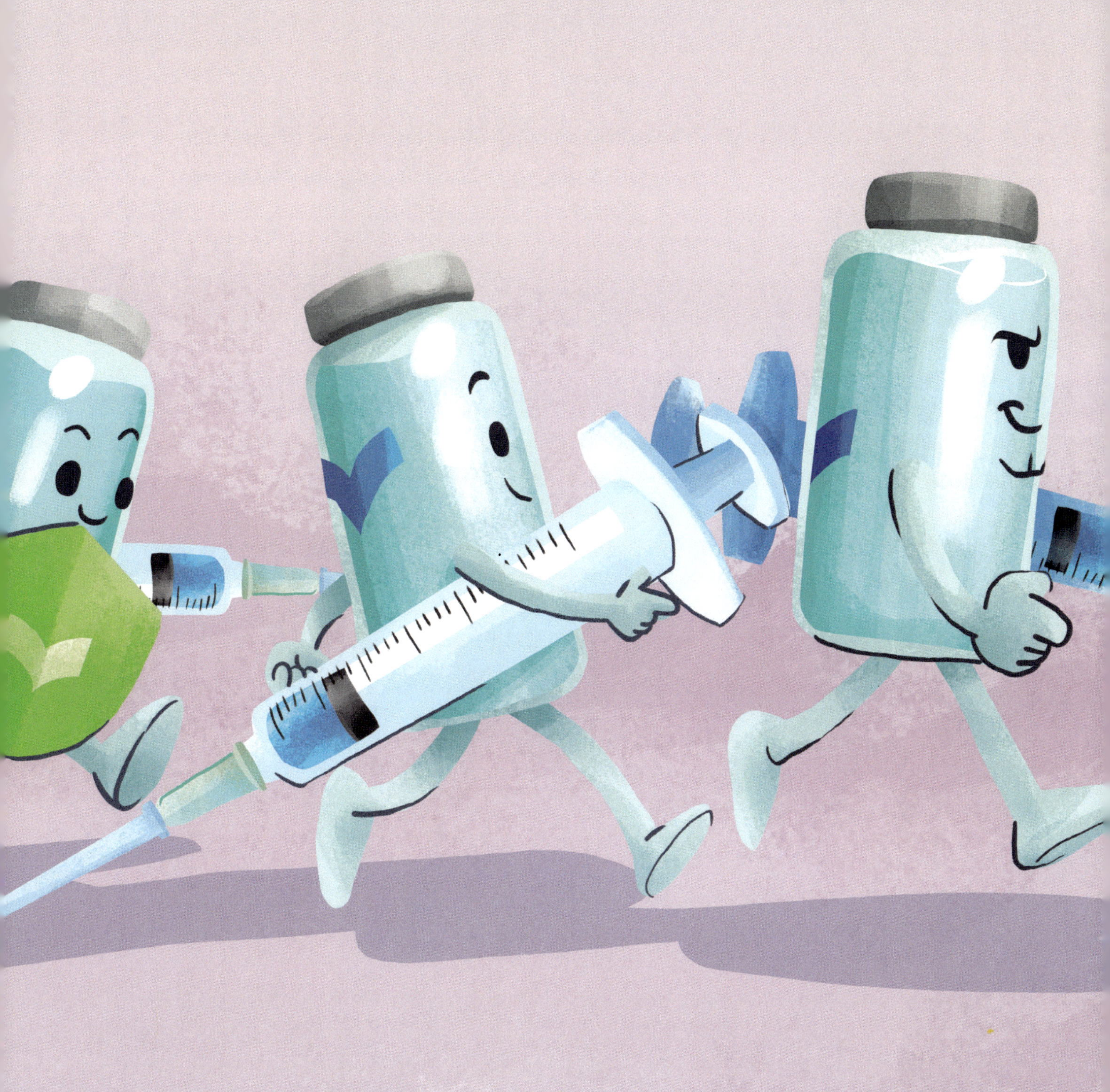

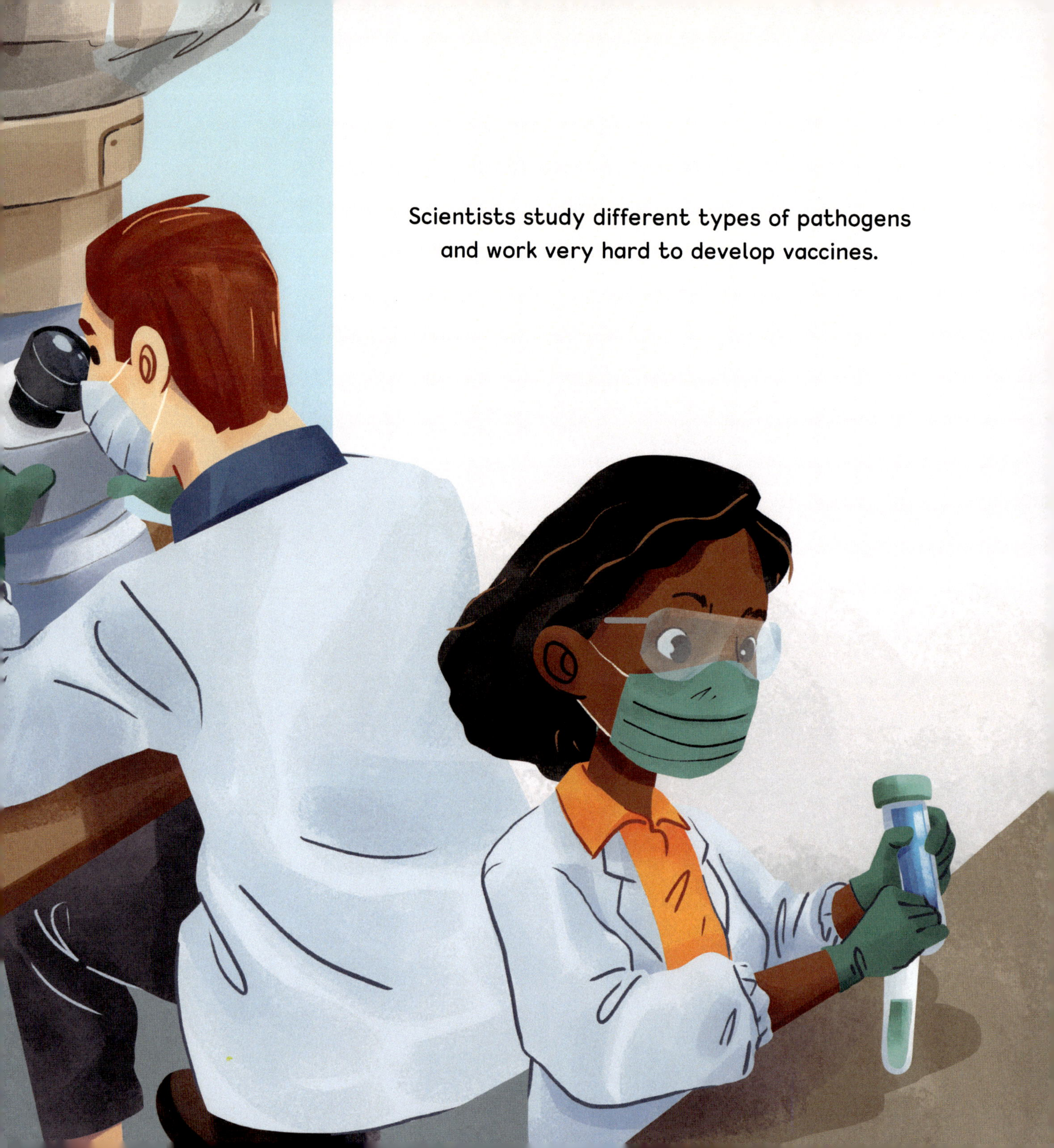

Scientists study different types of pathogens and work very hard to develop vaccines.

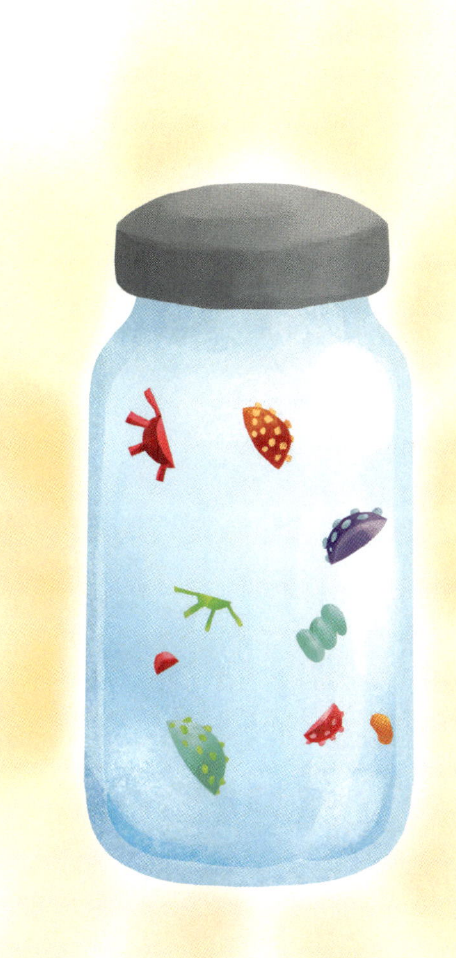

These vaccines are usually made from **ANTIGENS**,
tiny bits of germs that will turn your immune system on.

Your **IMMUNE SYSTEM** is your body's way of protecting itself from outside invaders. The vaccine will tell your immune system to go to work.

White Blood Cells
Group of cells that help protect your body from getting sick

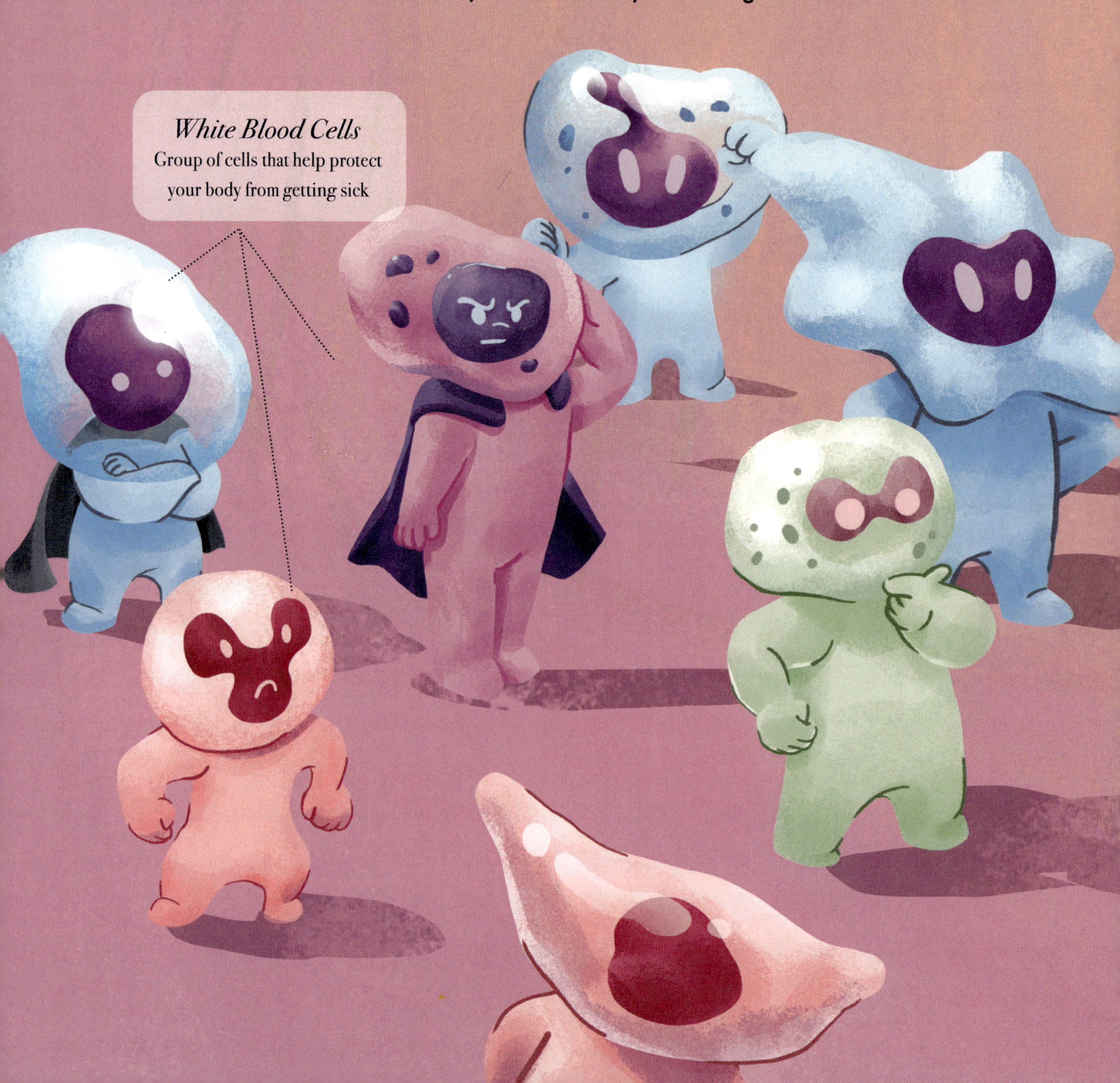

They show your body what these harmful germs look like and give it a practice round to fight them off.

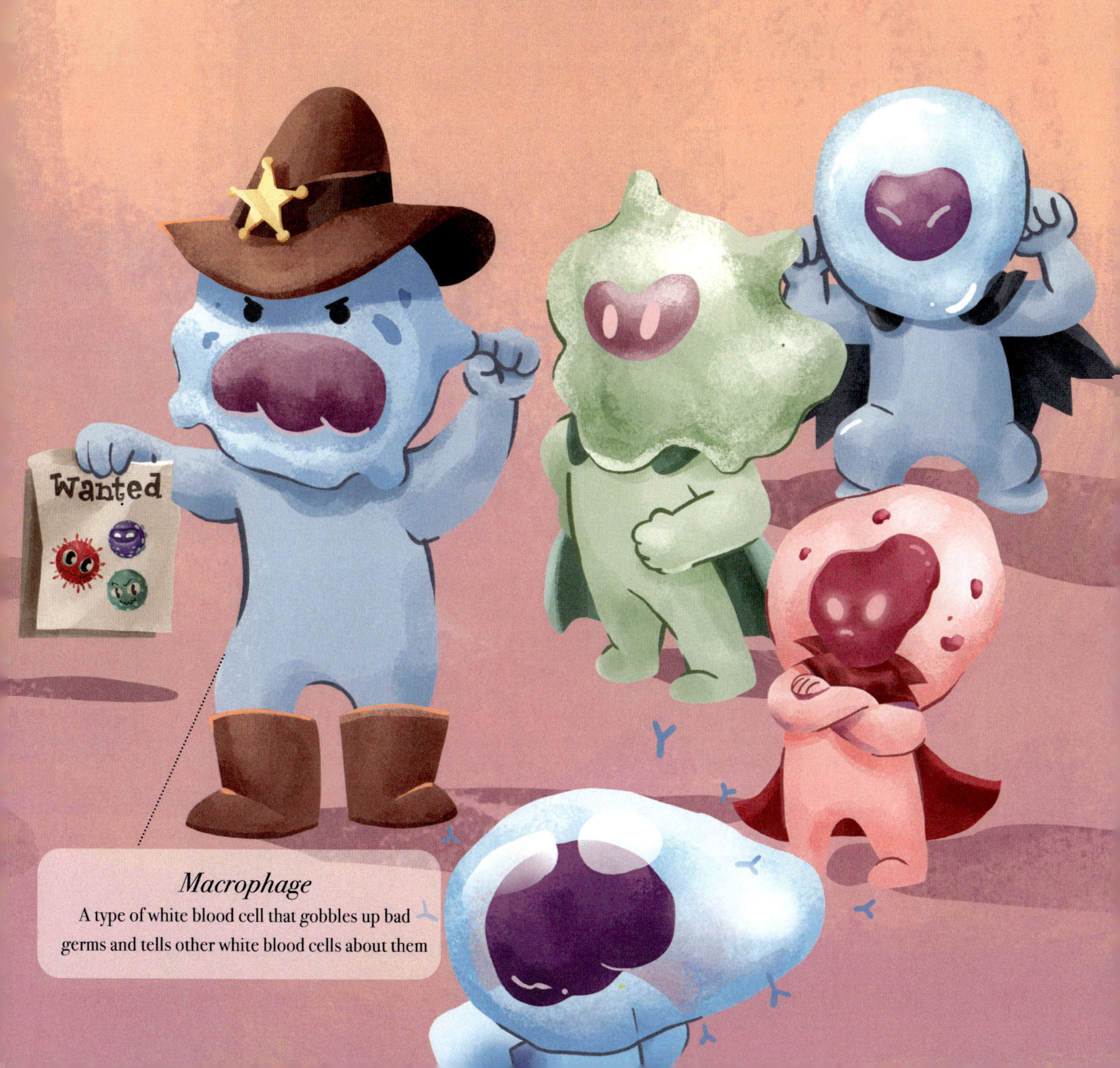

Macrophage
A type of white blood cell that gobbles up bad germs and tells other white blood cells about them

Your body then creates **ANTIBODIES**.

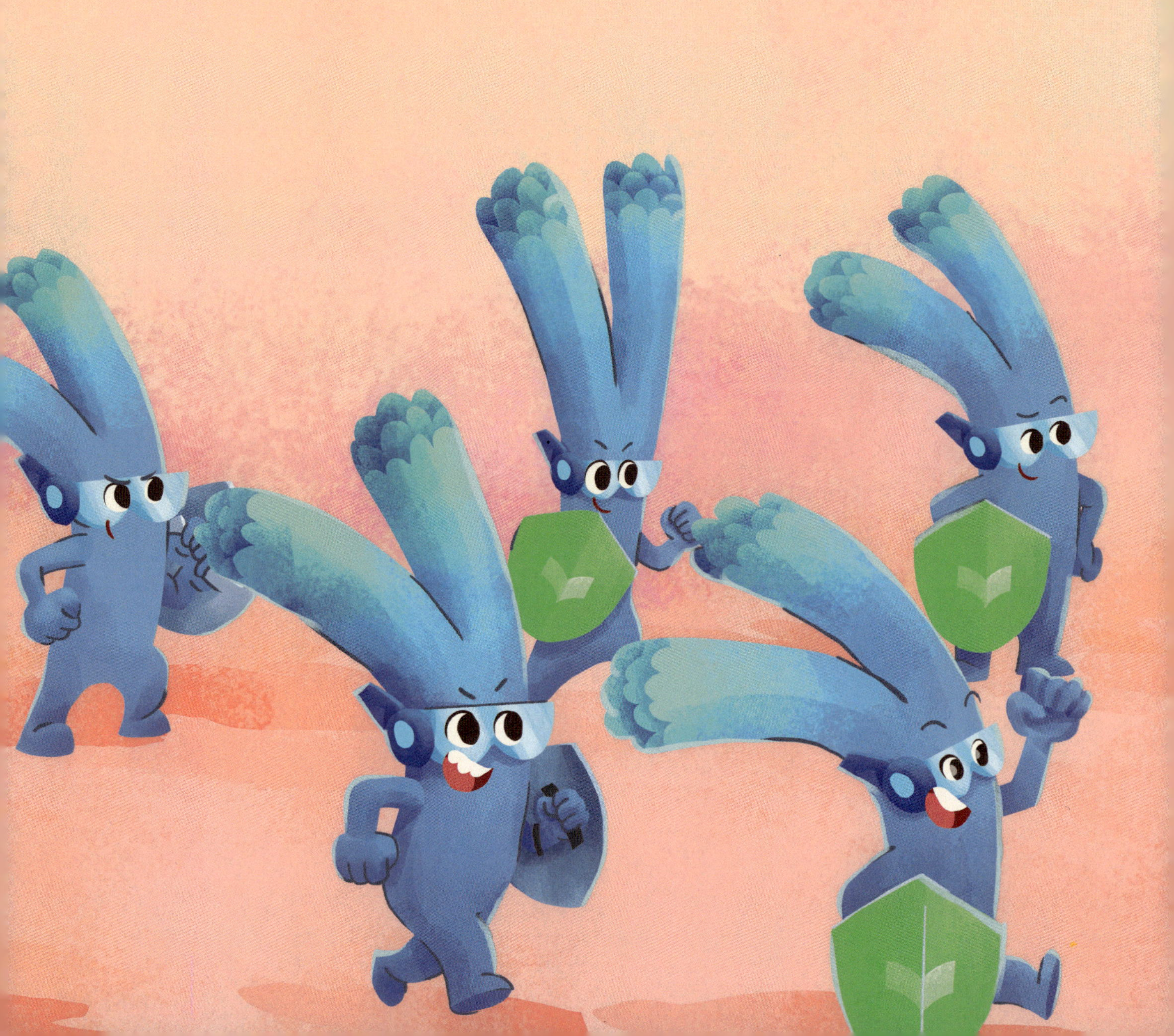

These are special defenders that will recognize the germs and protect you from them in the future.

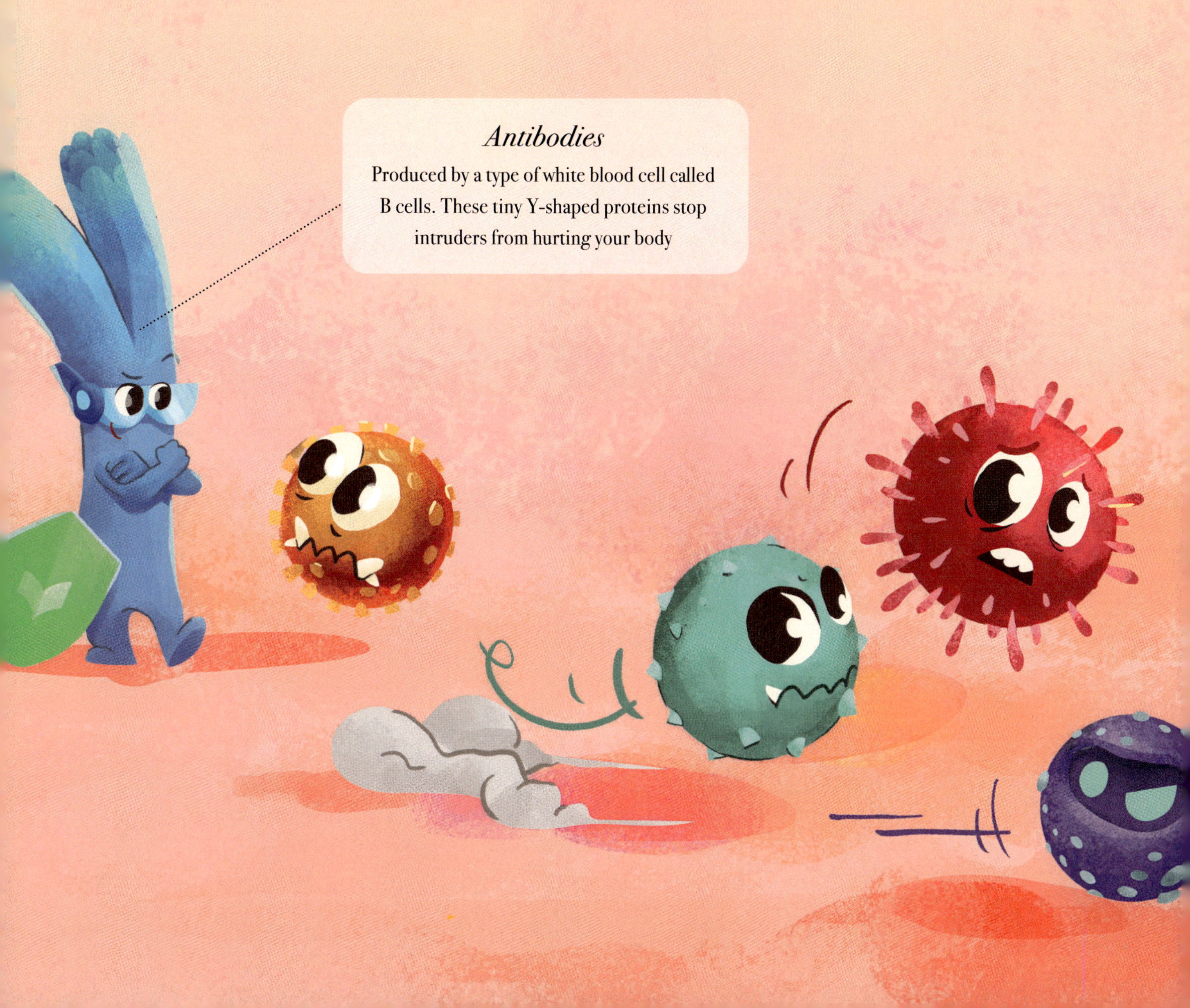

To put the vaccine into our bodies, a shot is usually given using a **SYRINGE**. It has a needle with a tiny hole on one end, a barrel in the middle containing medicine, and a plunger at the other end.

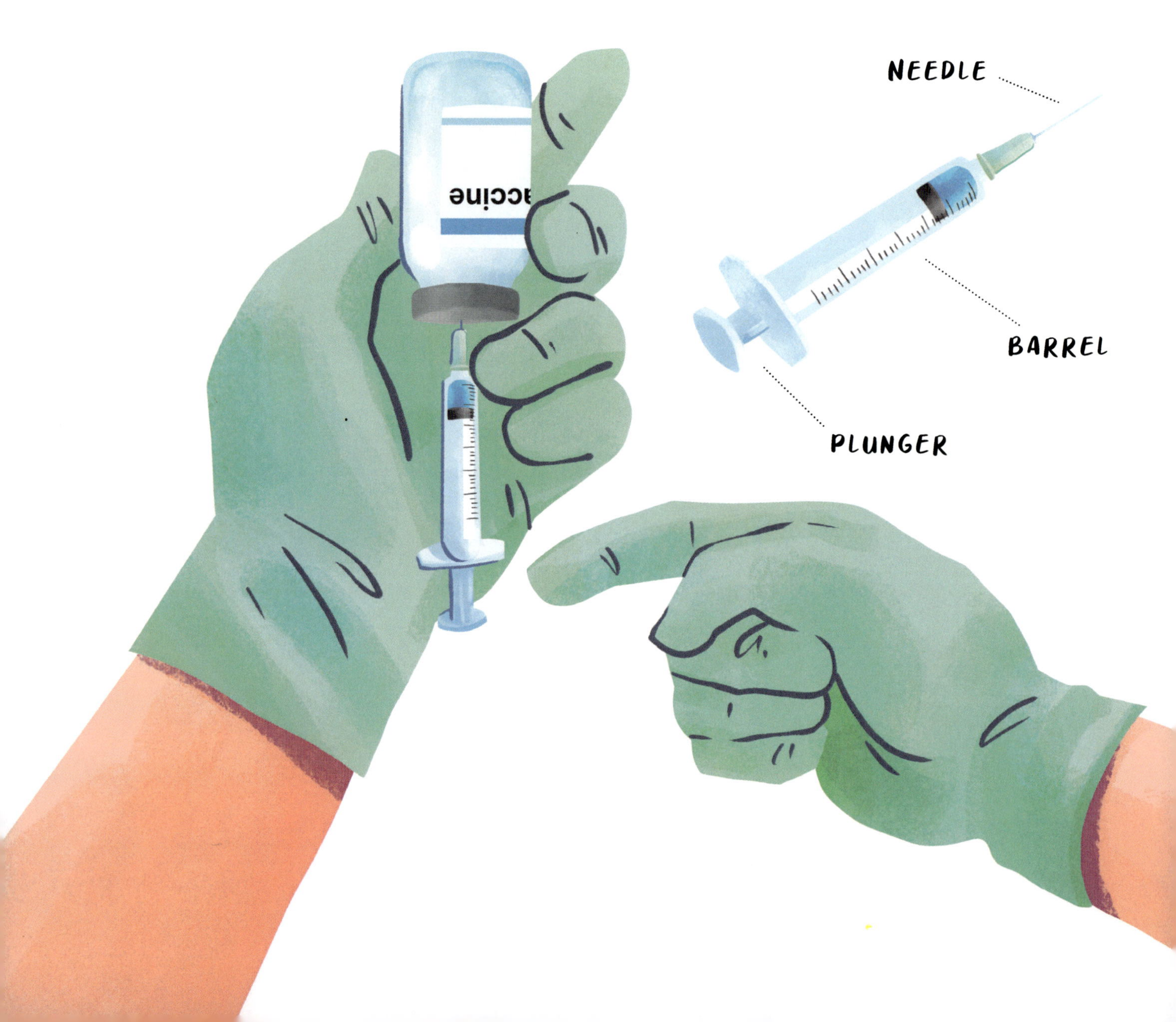

CLEAN SKIN

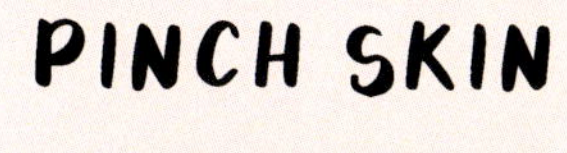

INJECT

1.

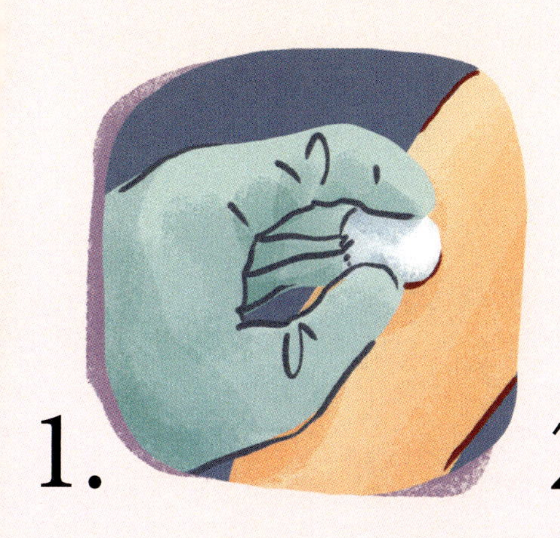

2.

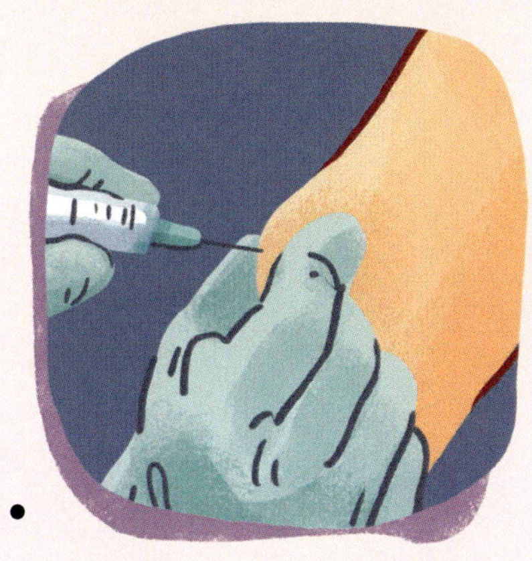

3.

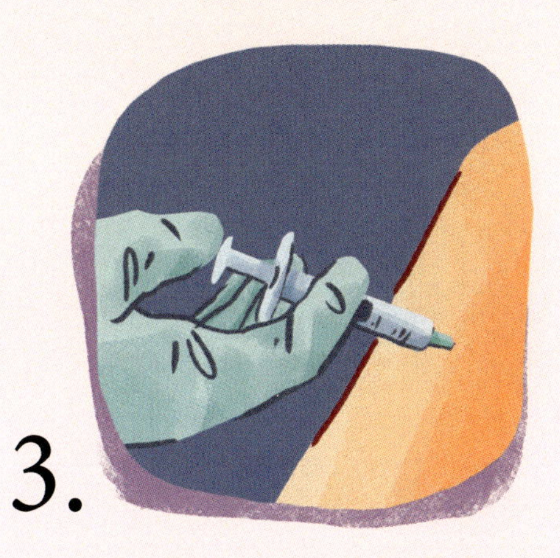

A doctor or nurse will insert the needle and press down on the plunger to inject the vaccine into your body.

It's important to stay relaxed and keep still so the medicine can travel easily.

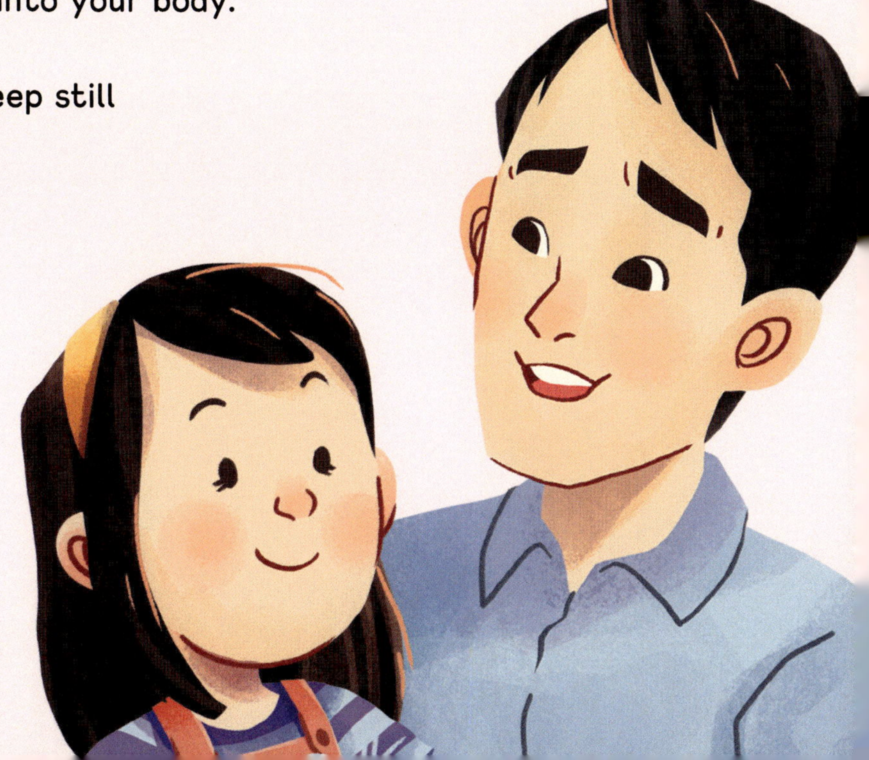

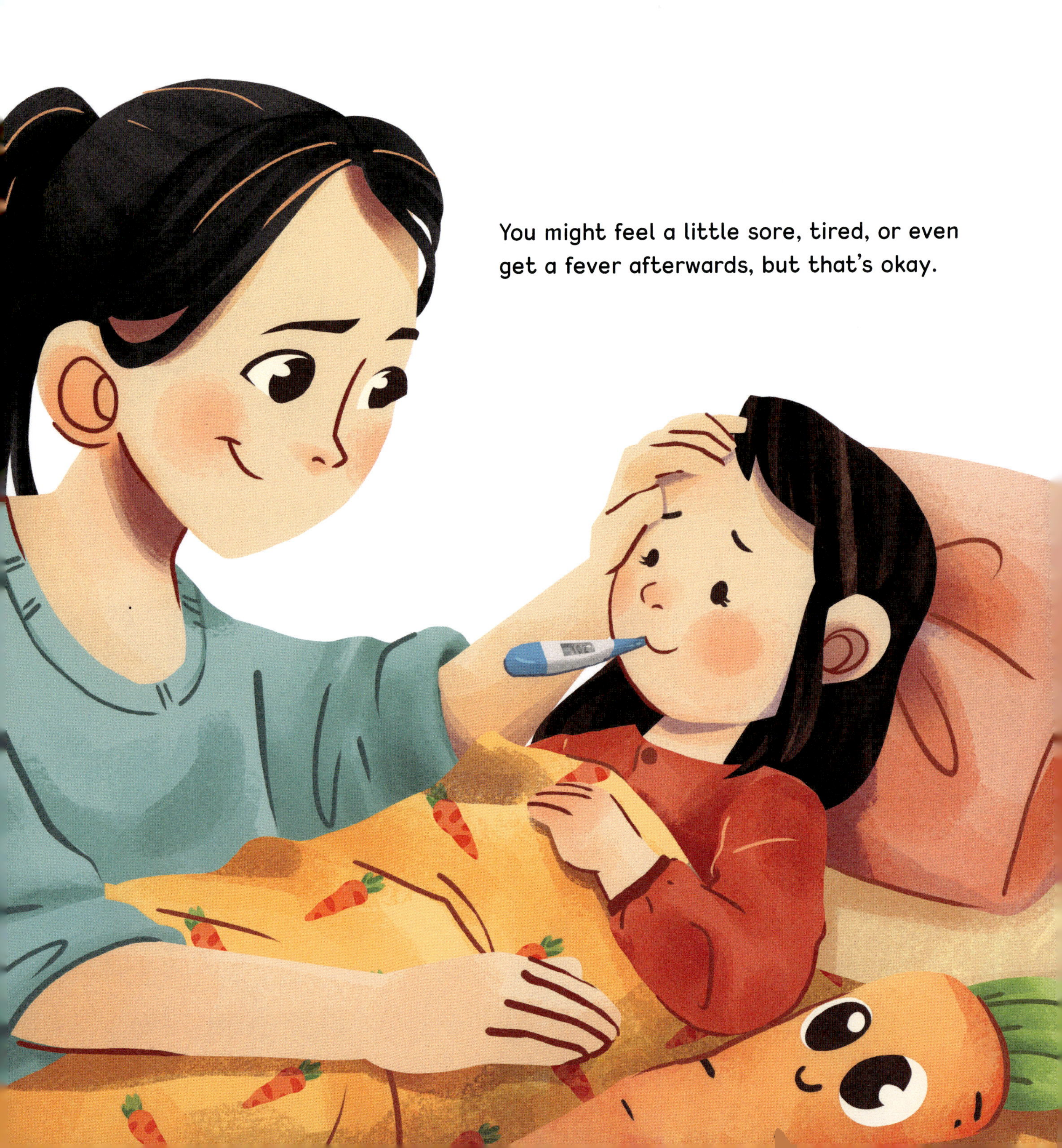

You might feel a little sore, tired, or even get a fever afterwards, but that's okay.

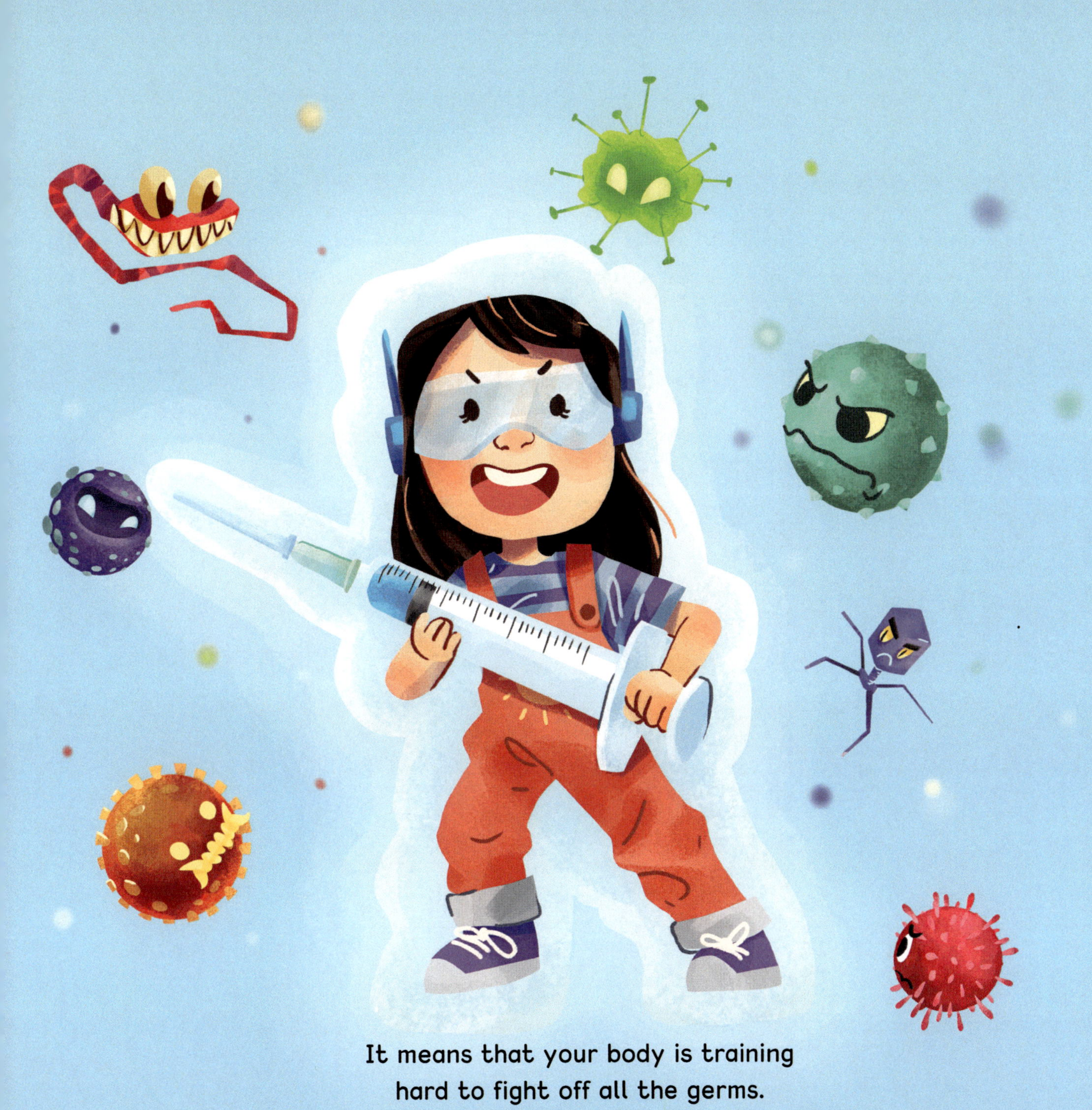

It means that your body is training
hard to fight off all the germs.

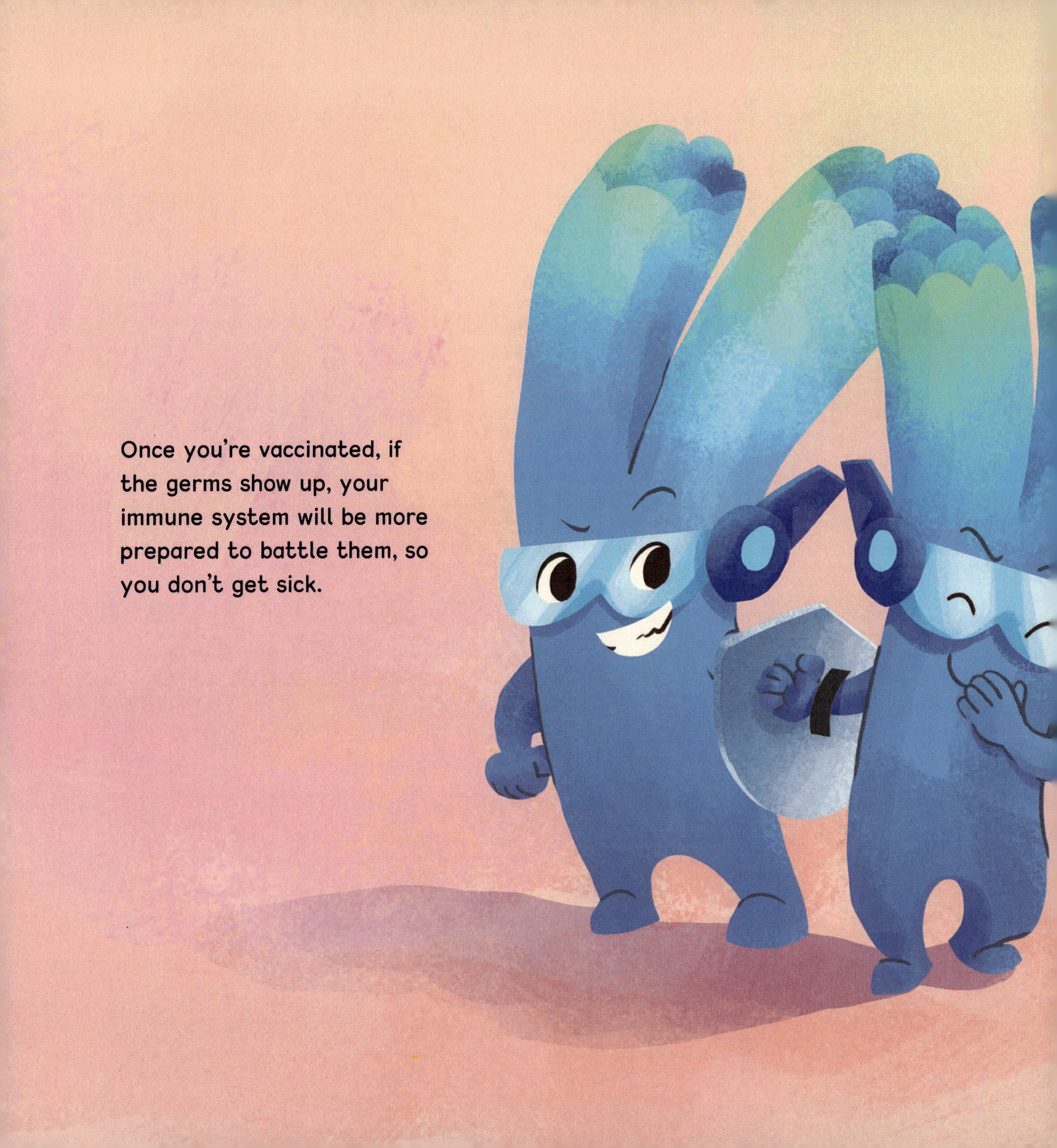

Once you're vaccinated, if the germs show up, your immune system will be more prepared to battle them, so you don't get sick.

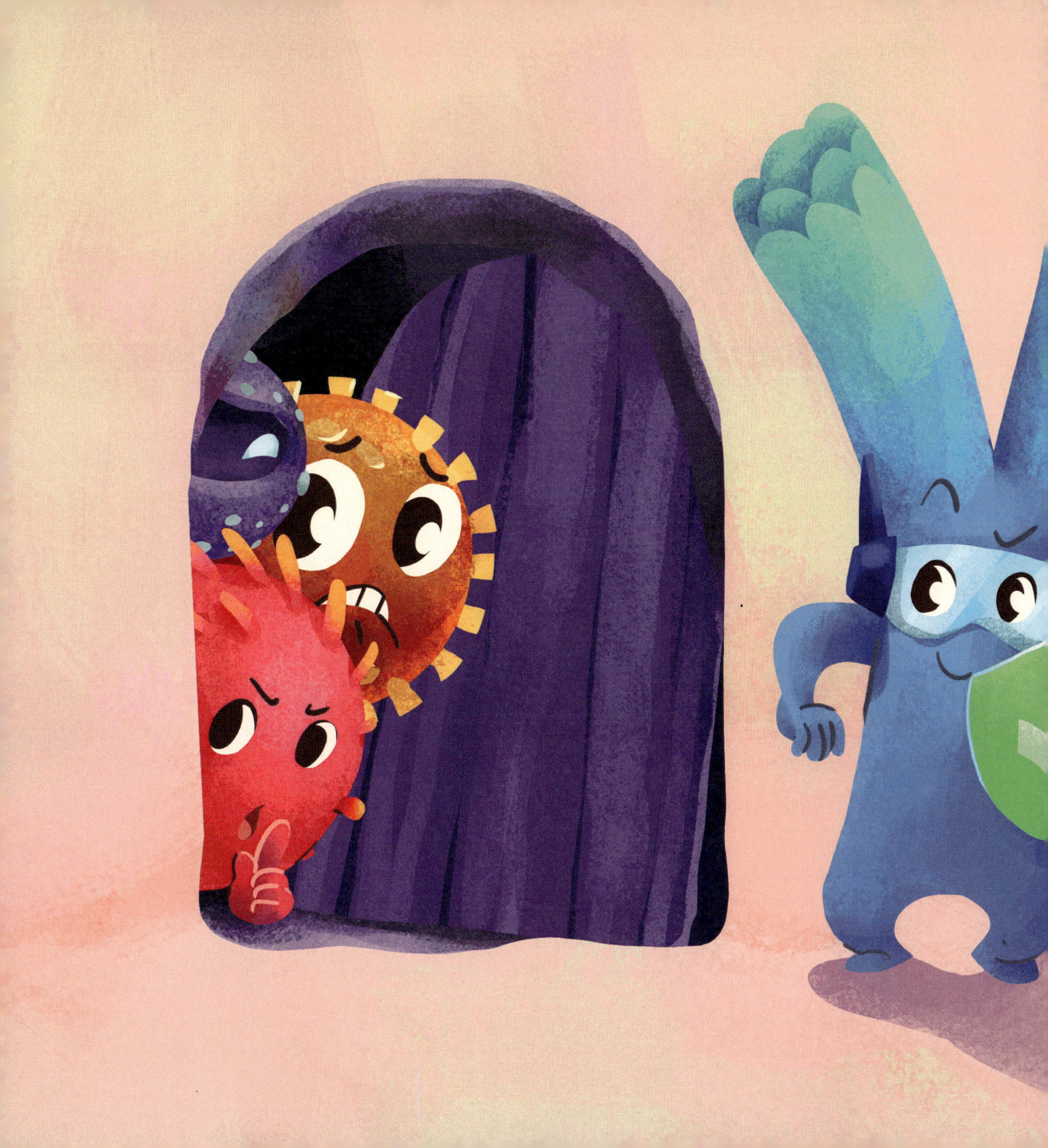

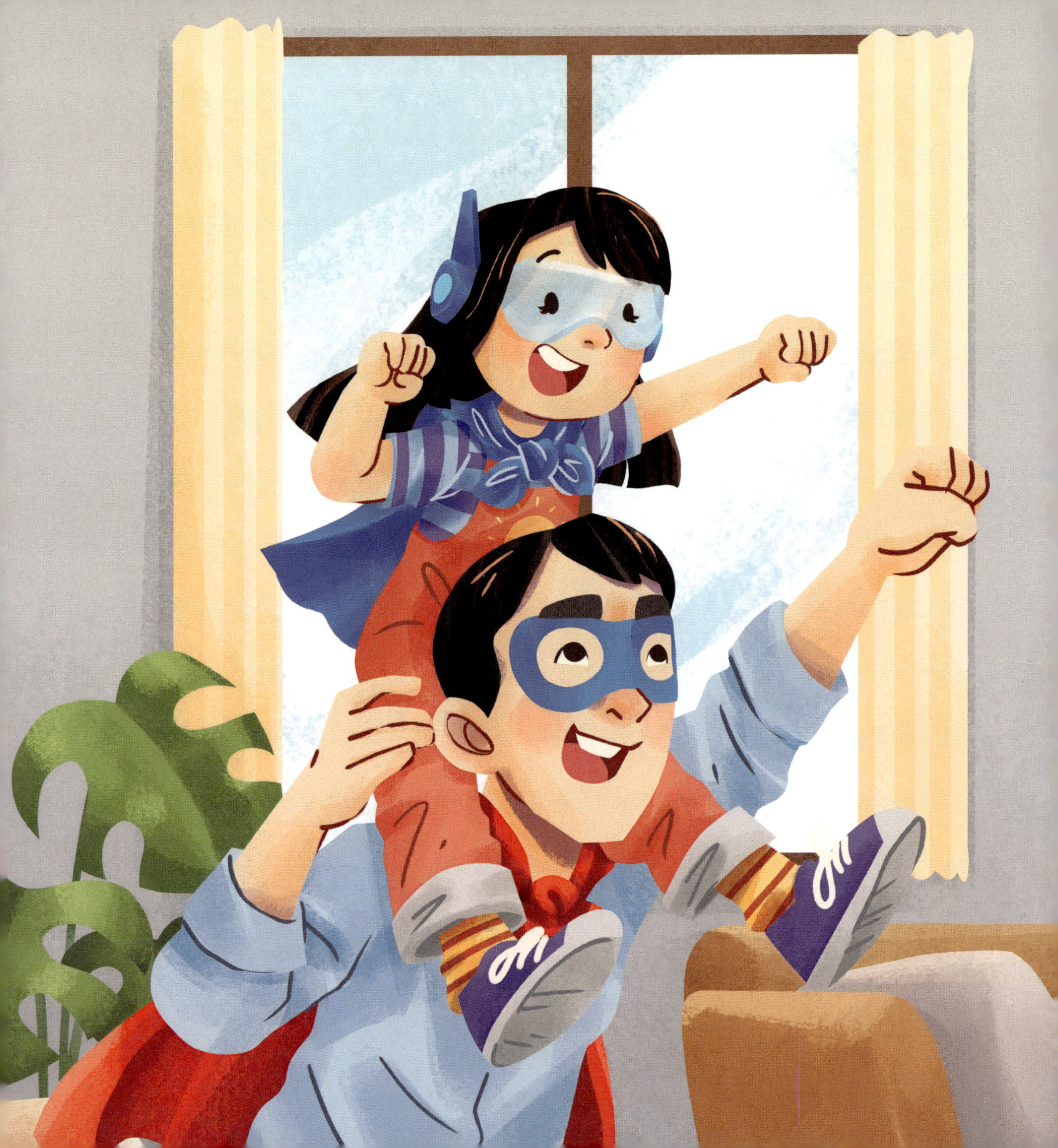

Now I get it! Vaccines will help my body make tiny defenders to battle germs and keep me healthy and strong.

That doesn't sound scary.
That actually sounds pretty COOL!

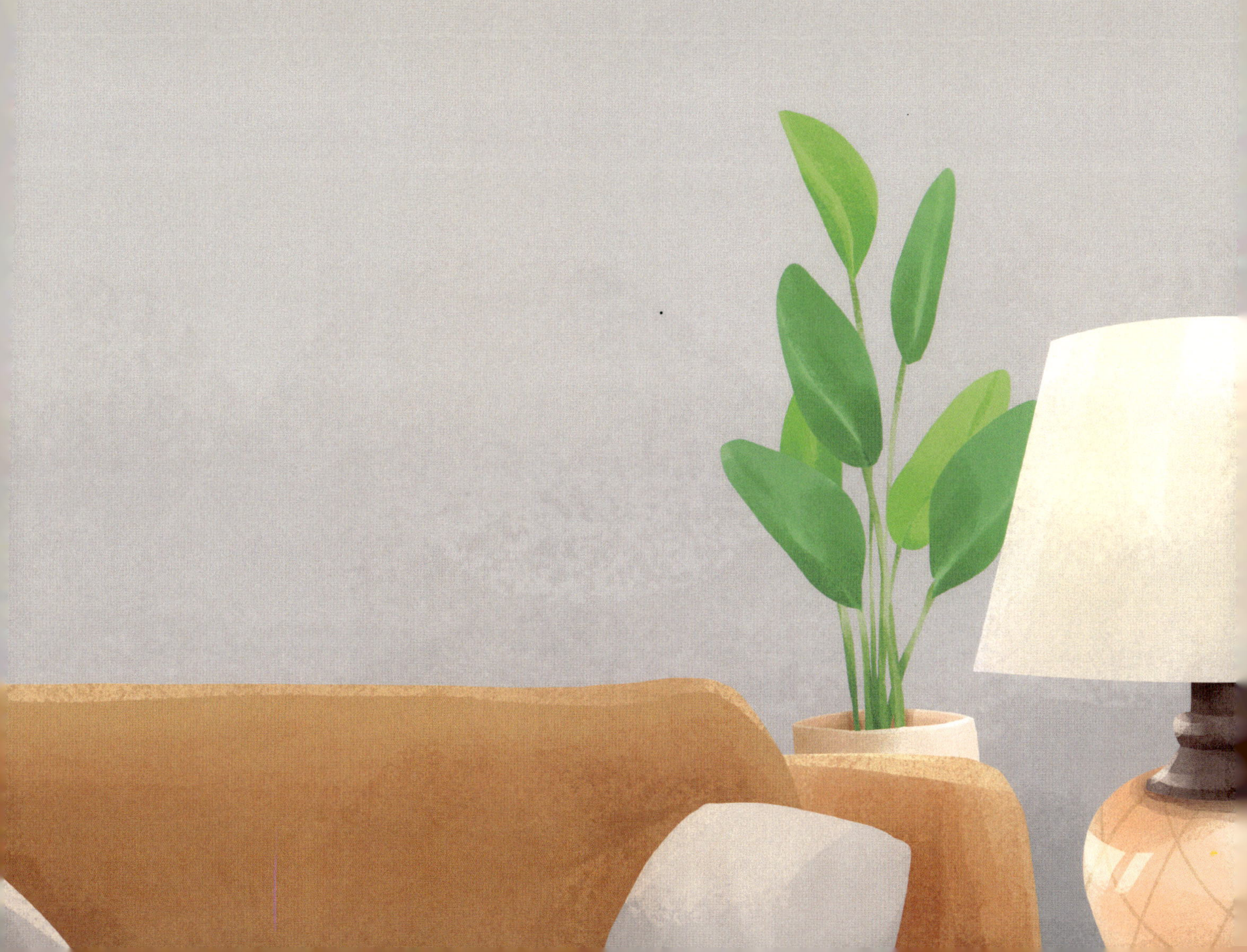

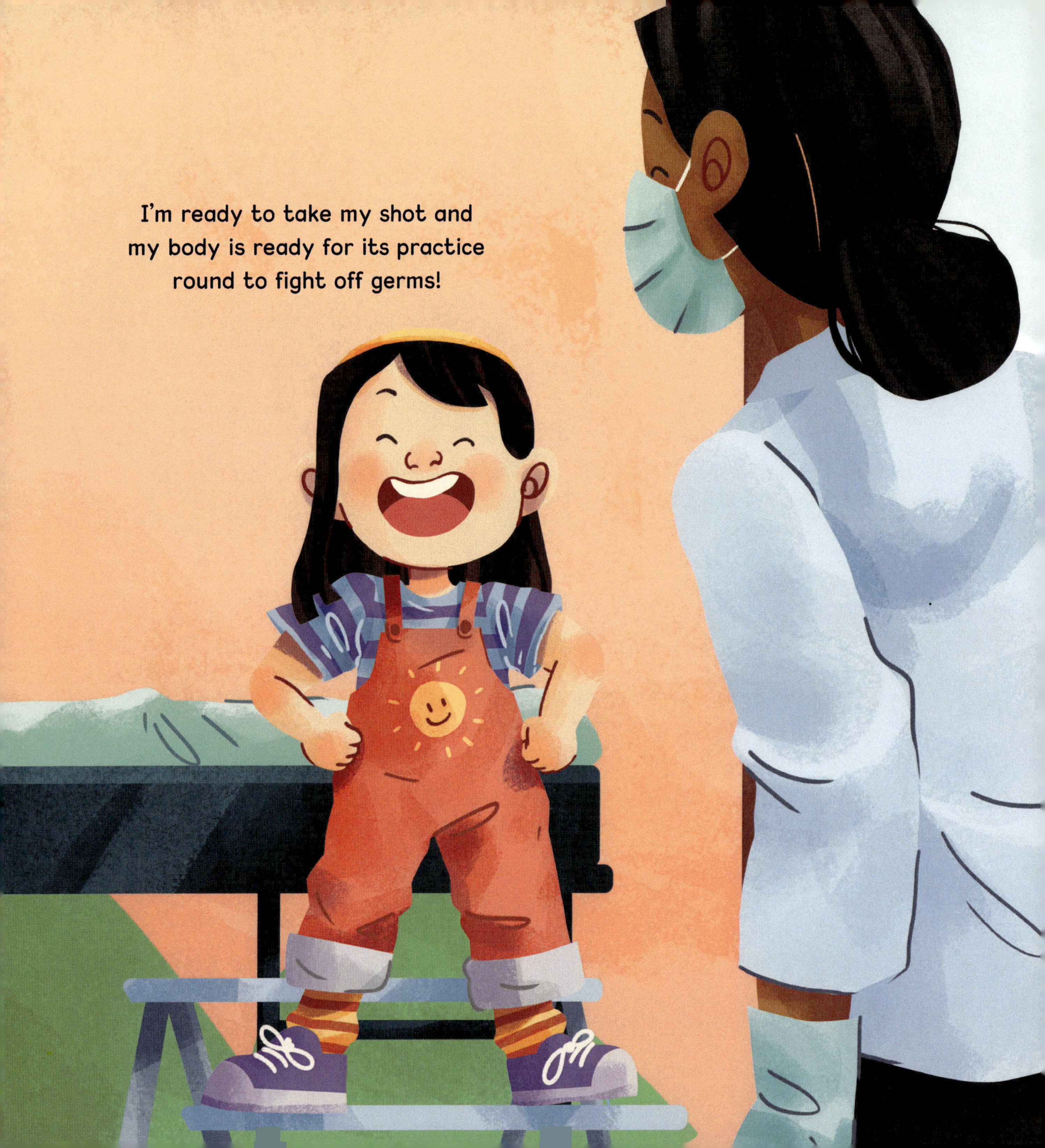

I'm ready to take my shot and
my body is ready for its practice
round to fight off germs!

Just relax your arm like a soft noodle.
Close your eyes and before you know it, it's all done!

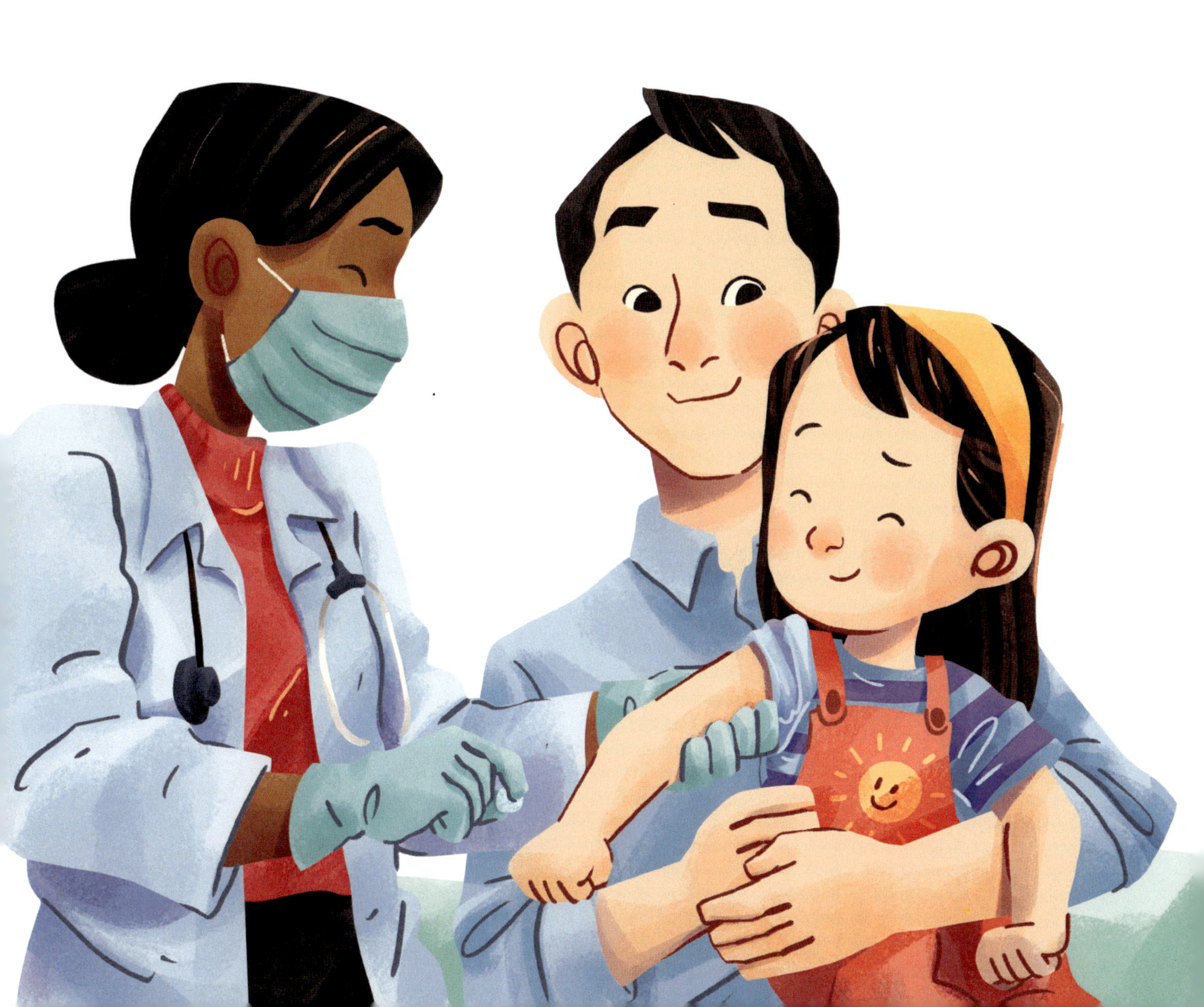

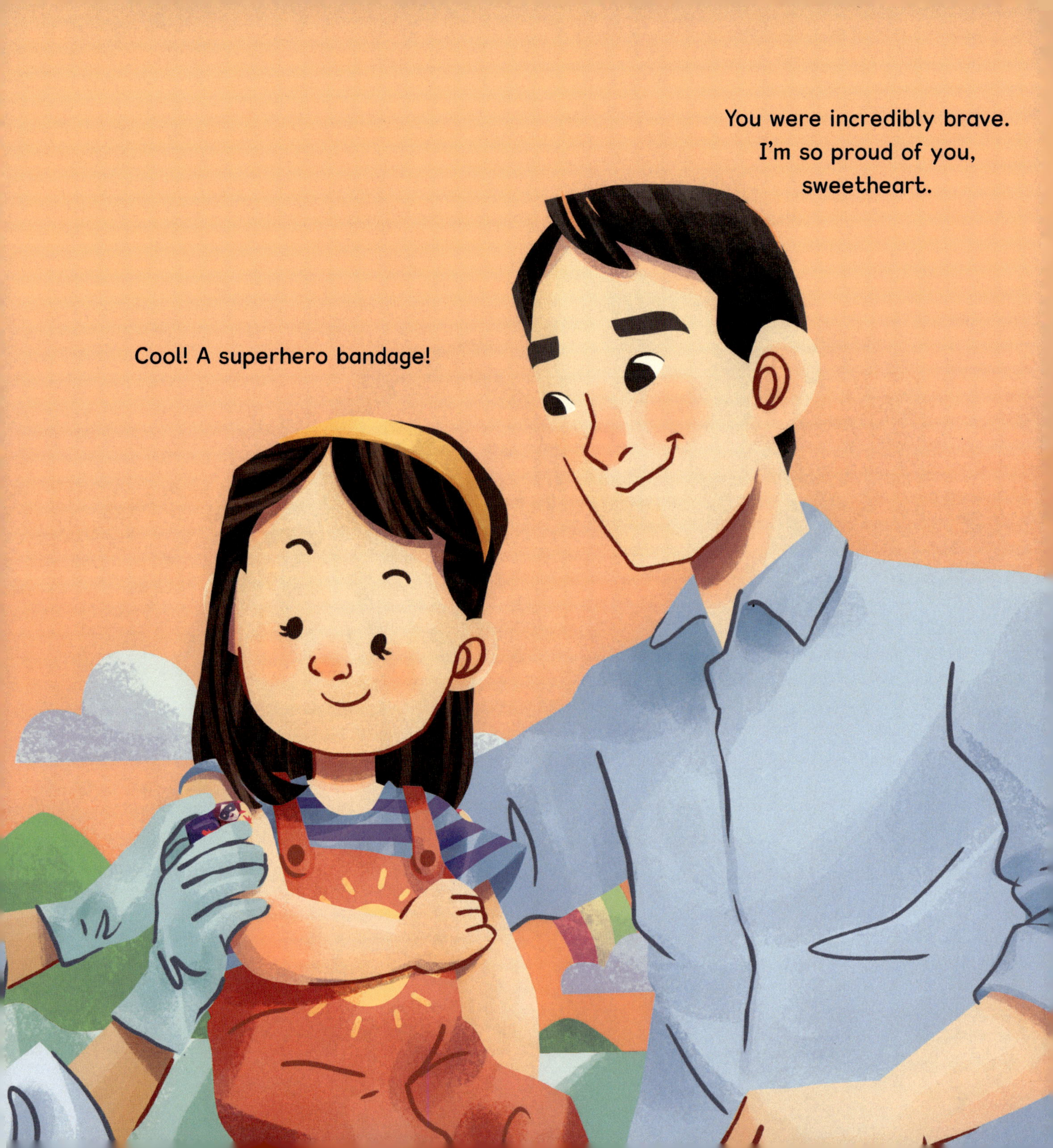
You were incredibly brave.
I'm so proud of you,
sweetheart.
Cool! A superhero bandage!

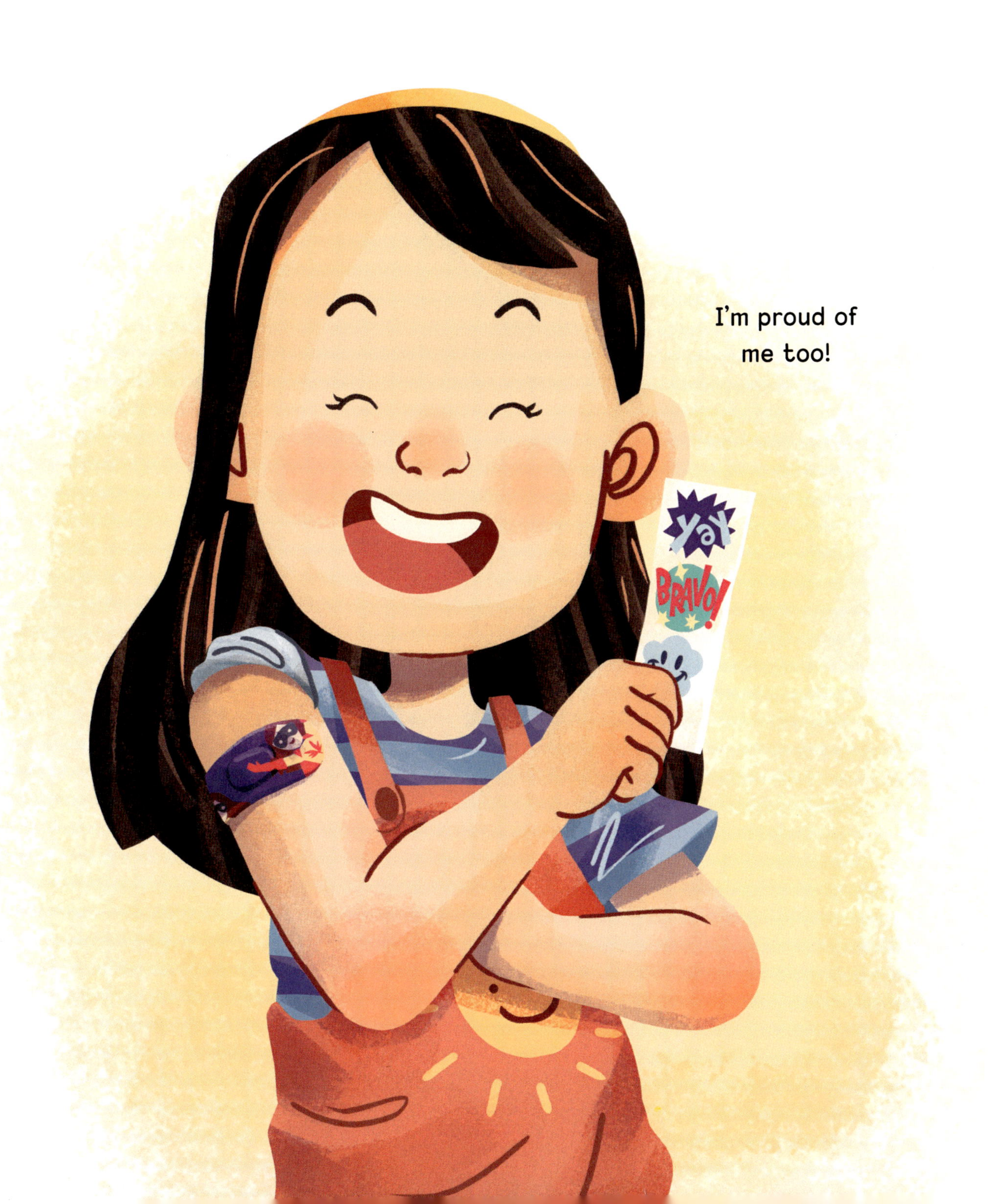

I’m proud of
me too!

Made in the USA
Las Vegas, NV
31 July 2024